# How to Get a Job in
# HEALTH CARE

# How to Get a Job in HEALTH CARE

SECOND EDITION

## Robert H. Zedlitz, M.A.

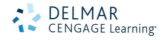

DELMAR
CENGAGE Learning®

Australia • Brazil • Japan • Korea • Mexico • Singapore • Spain • United Kingdom • United States

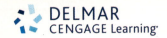

**How to Get a Job in Health Care, 2nd Ed.**
Robert H. Zedlitz, M.A.

Vice President, Careers and Computing:
Dave Garza

Director of Learning Solutions:
Matthew Kane

Senior Acquisitions Editor: Matt Seeley

Managing Editor: Marah Bellegarde

Senior Product Manager: Laura J. Wood

Editorial Assistant: Danielle Yannotti

Vice President, Marketing: Jennifer Ann Baker

Marketing Director: Wendy E. Mapstone

Senior Marketing Manager: Kristin McNary

Associate Marketing Manager:
Jonathan Sheehan

Senior Director, Education Production:
Wendy A. Troeger

Production Manager: Andrew Crouth

Senior Content Project Manager:
Kara A. DiCaterino

Senior Art Director: David Arsenault

Technology Project Manager: Patricia Allen

For product information and technology assistance, contact us at
**Cengage Learning Customer & Sales Support, 1-800-354-9706**

For permission to use material from this text or product,
submit all requests online at **www.cengage.com/permissions**.
Further permissions questions can be e-mailed to
**permissionrequest@cengage.com**

Library of Congress Control Number: 2011942792

ISBN-13: 978-1-1116-4008-8

ISBN-10: 1-1116-4008-4

**Delmar**
5 Maxwell Drive
Clifton Park, NY 12065-2919
USA

Cengage Learning is a leading provider of customized learning solutions with office locations around the globe, including Singapore, the United Kingdom, Australia, Mexico, Brazil, and Japan. Locate your local office at:
**international.cengage.com/region**

Cengage Learning products are represented in Canada by
Nelson Education, Ltd.

To learn more about Delmar, visit **www.cengage.com/delmar**

Purchase any of our products at your local college store or at our preferred online store **www.cengagebrain.com**

**Notice to the Reader**

Publisher does not warrant or guarantee any of the products described herein or perform any independent analysis in connection with any of the product information contained herein. Publisher does not assume, and expressly disclaims, any obligation to obtain and include information other than that provided to it by the manufacturer. The reader is expressly warned to consider and adopt all safety precautions that might be indicated by the activities described herein and to avoid all potential hazards. By following the instructions contained herein, the reader willingly assumes all risks in connection with such instructions. The publisher makes no representations or warranties of any kind, including but not limited to, the warranties of fitness for particular purpose or merchantability, nor are any such representations implied with respect to the material set forth herein, and the publisher takes no responsibility with respect to such material. The publisher shall not be liable for any special, consequential, or exemplary damages resulting, in whole or part, from the readers' use of, or reliance upon, this material.

Printed in the United States of America
1 2 3 4 5 6 7 16 15 14 13 12

# Contents

| | |
|---|---|
| **Preface** | **vii** |
| **Acknowledgments** | **xv** |
| **Introduction to Students** | **xvii** |
| **Using This Text and StudyWARE™ with ResGen Software** | **1** |
| Understanding the Icons | 1 |
| Using StudyWARE™ with ResGen | 1 |

| | |
|---|---|
| **Section 1: Getting and Starting a Job in Health Care** | **7** |
| Introduction | 7 |
| **Step 1** Health Care Resume | 9 |
| **Step 2** Health Care Cover Letter | 22 |
| **Step 3** Health Care Employment Application | 30 |
| **Step 4** Finding and Researching a Health Care Job and Facility | 36 |
| **Step 5** How to Prepare for a Health Care Interview | 47 |
| **Step 6** During the Health Care Interview | 57 |
| **Step 7** After the Health Care Interview | 65 |
| **Step 8** How to Start a Health Care Job | 72 |

| | |
|---|---|
| **Section 2: Leaving a Health Care Job … Gracefully** | **79** |
| Introduction | 79 |
| **Step 1** Questions to Consider Before Leaving a Health Care Job | 80 |
| **Step 2** The Best Way to Leave a Health Care Job | 84 |
| **Step 3** Health Care Reference Letter | 89 |

## Section 3: Getting, Starting, and Leaving a Job in Health Care—Activities

**97**

Introduction    97

1. Checklist of Employment Power Words and Phrases    99

2. Writing Health Care Job Objectives    101

3. Constructing a Health Care Resume    103

    3-1    Standard Resume (Practice Sheet)    103

    3-2    Chronological Resume (Practice Sheet)    105

    3-3    Functional Resume (Practice Sheet)    107

    3-4    Combination Resume (Practice Sheet)    109

4. Constructing a Health Care Reference List    111

5. Writing a Health Care Cover Letter    113

6. Completing a Health Care Employment Application    115

7. Finding Health Care Job Leads    121

8. Researching a Health Care Facility    125

9-1 Answering Interview Questions    129

9-2 Practice Interview Evaluation Form    133

10. Health Care Case Study Questions    135

11. Preparing a Health Care Post-Interview Letter    139

12. Identifying Health Care Personal Qualities    141

13. Health Care Case Study—Decision Time    143

14. Writing a Health Care Resignation Letter    145

15. Health Care Exit Conversation    147

16. Constructing a Health Care Reference Letter    149

## Message from the Author, Robert Zedlitz

*Work-based learning, school to work, work experience education,* and *linked learning* are terms that define my educational approach during my years instructing students. My goal was to teach job-search skills to obtain not just any job but the job you deserve and to make the process less perplexing. As a facilitator between students and employers, I prepared students for what their employers wanted and expected. With these elements my first job process kit was published. What was vague to the job seeker became clear-cut. Introspection, job research, and promoting one's employability was placed in the job seeker's hands.

Early in my career, I met with then Secretary of Labor, Willard Wirtz, when he spoke in the San Francisco Bay area on his strategy of integrating the worlds of school and work. Wirtz was a proponent of the job process I used, and inscribed in my copy of his book, *The Boundless Resource,* "For Bob Zedlitz: With great admiration for what he is doing." Since then I have continued my quest for refining the employment process, and my journey has led me to this second edition of *How to Get a Job in Health Care.*

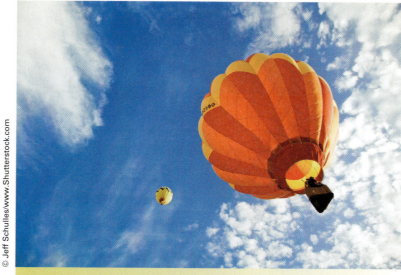

© Jeff Schulles/www.Shutterstock.com

**Reach for your dream job in health care.**

*How to Get a Job in Health Care* provides an easy-to-follow, step-by-step guide for obtaining the job you want in the health care industry. It offers an employment process, materials, and techniques that develop your professional image and elevate your confidence level in obtaining employment. *How to Get a Job in Health Care* even gives you strategies to ensure that you start your new job successfully. In addition, it offers a graceful method to use when changing a health care position.

This manual is for you if you are:

- Ready to start your health care career
- Making a health care job change
- Changing careers to go into health care
- Laid off or downsized

# How This Text Is Organized

*How to Get a Job in Health Care* is an employment manual divided into three sections. Sections 1 and 2 cover how to get, start, and leave a job, while Section 3 activities provide documents necessary for success in the health care job process. Individualized material allows you to progress at your own pace. At the beginning of each step in Sections 1 and 2, a summary of its important features provides a quick review and guide to the contents.

*How to Get a Job in Health Care*, your personal guide, is vital to success in gaining employment. You will have the advantage of being prepared because you will have acquired the employment manual, and copies of important employment documents, saved in an employment portfolio and as files to your personal thumb drive. You will be able to reference the manual and update the documents to use throughout your health care career.

**Note:** The website addresses referred to in *How to Get a Job in Health Care* were current when this manual was published.

## Section 1: Getting and Starting a Job in Health Care

Section 1 of the manual, which contains 8 steps with activities, forms an effective, workable guide for actually landing the position, as well as tips to get you off to a good start in your health care career.

## Section 2: Leaving a Health Care Job … Gracefully

Section 2 of *How to Get a Job in Health Care* contains 3 steps with valuable advice and insight concerning how to leave a health care job gracefully with excellent references. There is far more to leaving a job than saying, "I quit." This section includes procedures and activities that will end your job on a positive note.

## Section 3: Getting, Starting, and Leaving a Job in Health Care—Activities

Section 3 of this manual contains self-directed activities to complete each step of Section 1 and Section 2. The instructions in Sections 1 and 2 are reinforced by 16 self-directed, meaningful activities that allow you to participate while being led systematically through the text. The activities make *How to Get a Job in Health Care* action orientated.

The following activities are included:

Activity 1 Checklist of Employment Power Words and Phrases

Activity 2 Writing Health Care Job Objectives

Activity 3 Constructing a Health Care Resume

Activity 4 Constructing a Health Care Reference List

Activity 5 Writing a Health Care Cover Letter

Activity 6 Completing a Health Care Employment Application

Activity 7 Finding Health Care Job Leads

Activity 8 Researching a Health Care Facility

Activity 9 Answering Interview Questions and Practice Interview Evaluation Form

Activity 10 Health Care Case Study Questions

Activity 11 Preparing a Health Care Post-Interview Letter

Activity 12 Identifying Health Care Personal Qualities

Activity 13 Health Care Case Study—Decision Time

Activity 14 Writing a Health Care Resignation Letter

Activity 15 Health Care Exit Conversation

Activity 16 Constructing a Health Care Reference Letter

PORTFOLIO
UPDATE

## Employment Portfolio

As each activity in Section 3 of *How to Get a Job in Health Care* is completed, including those keyed on the software, and resumes and employment letters created by your Resume Generator, a copy can be placed in an employment portfolio. The employment portfolio can be any type of your choosing. It can be as simple as a file folder which establishes a record of valuable papers necessary for employment in the health care industry. Your employment portfolio will provide guidelines for securing and leaving jobs now and in your future health care career. An employment portfolio containing all of these materials will be extremely convenient in the future, when easy access to these employment aids is needed. Throughout the text, the icon shown here in the margin will appear as a reminder to place activities, resumes, and letters into your employment portfolio.

# New to Second Edition—Overview of Content Changes

The author understands that employment documents are a necessary key for your health care career success. This edition provides four new resume styles that describe a variety of health care applicant qualifications. Updated health care letters include:

- Cover letters to create a good first impression
- Post-interview thank-you letter and note card exhibit strong desire
- Reference letter to gain future employment
- Resignation letter to end your job in a positive, mature way

Unique health care job search techniques to advance your potential include:

- Business card for employer and network contacts
- Thank-you note and e-mail message make a positive impact
- Thirty-second pitch makes an emphatic contact

You will find employer job leads online, research and advance your health care career on O*Net OnLine, and research a health care employer before an interview. In addition to getting and leaving a job, this edition includes a step for starting your health care job with:

- Tips for starting off as a professional
- How to ace your performance review
- How positive personal qualities count
- Advice to help you advance in your heath care job and career

*How to Get a Job in Health Care* is now a complete employment resource for your health care career.

# New to Second Edition—Specific Changes

All steps include new, full-color photographs with descriptive captions that highlight everything from appropriate dress to eye contact and interview skills. A new full-color text design provides a highly inviting pedagogy to enhance understanding of the concepts discussed. Other content-specific changes are:

## Section 1

### Step 1

- New examples of four types of resumes including standard, chronological, functional, and combination resumes, and a new reference list example which coordinates with the standard resume.

- Updated content related to electronic resumes and using professional personal e-mail addresses.

## Step 2

- New cover letter example with others revised and updated, tips for cover letter headings, and updated newspaper ads.

- New photographs show how skills learned in school relate to health care employment.

## Step 3

- New employment application example.

- New content about creating online accounts with potential employers in order to track the job application process.

## Step 4

- Updated and new content on finding and preparing for job leads, including: networking, creating business cards and thank-you notes, using a mentor, contacting employers and conducting market research, and utilizing newspaper and Internet job listings.

- New information on questions to answer before an interview, including how to research a job using O*Net Online.

## Step 5

- Expanded content on preparing for an interview, including possible interview questions and responses.

- New section on Getting Answers to Your Employment Questions and what questions to get answered before accepting a health care job offer.

- New section on Interview Killer Questions and what not to ask at a job interview.

- A new activity provides a Practice Interview Evaluation Form to help role-play and evaluate performance in a mock interview.

## Step 6

- Revised and updated model interview scenario including how to describe a stressful situation.

- Expanded content on appropriate closing remarks at an interview, including follow-up questions to ask and last ways to sell yourself to a potential employer.

## Step 7

- Expanded content about writing a post-interview letter, including a checklist for what to include in the letter.

- Examples of a handwritten interview follow-up note and e-mail for a hiring decision.

- New section on how to follow up after a health care interview in order to find out about a hiring decision.

### Step 8

- New! This new step describes how to start a job in health care and includes a procedure for acing a performance review. It also includes an activity related to identifying health care personal qualities and work styles using O*Net OnLine information.

## Section 2

### Step 1

- New photographs on considering advantages and disadvantages of a job change and learning new skills in order to set new health care career goals.

### Step 2

- Redesigned and updated resignation letter example.

- Tips for giving a positive reason for leaving a health care job.

- New photographs on presenting a resignation letter to a health care employer and planning an exit conversation.

### Step 3

- New reference letter example.

- New information on obtaining a reference letter from an employer and instructor.

- New section related to how to get the best outcome from being fired.

# Using the StudyWARE™ with ResGen Software

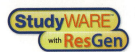

Icons like the one shown here in the margin indicate when it is time to use the accompanying software. Your software contains files you may use to supplement your *How to Get a Job in Health Care* activities and create your final resume and letter documents. After you draft selected activity worksheets in Section 3, you may use your personal software to edit these documents. The following sample documents are included in the software:

Standard Resume, Chronological Resume, Functional Resume, Combination Resume, Reference List, Cover Letters, Post-Interview Letter, Resignation Letter, and Reference Letter.

Your software also includes the Health Care Resume Generator. After you enter your personal data, this easy-to-use software will generate a variety of personalized employment documents designed specifically to help you find career success in the health care field.

As you work through *How to Get a Job in Health Care*, you are encouraged to save all of your keyed resume and letter files to your hard drive or thumb drive for future reference. You will be able to instantly use and easily update your employment documents.

See p. 1, Using this Text and StudyWARE™ with ResGen Software, for more information about the software.

# Instructor Support Materials

## Instructor Resources CD-ROM to Accompany *How to Get a Job in Health Care* ISBN-13: 978-1-111-64009-5

In addition to the students' materials, an Instructor's CD-ROM with valuable health care information is available to you, the educator. The *Instructor Resources CD-ROM to accompany How to Get a Job in Health Care* contains detailed strategies that help students complete the activities provided in this manual. There are helpful suggestions for teaching each part of the student's manual. Other strategies ensure that the student is thoroughly prepared for the health care industry employment process. These points include how to effectively:

- Present a resume to a prospective health care employer
- Write health care job objectives
- Read a health care employment advertisement
- Understand various health care employment applications
- Give positive or neutral reasons for leaving a health care job
- Answer the salary question
- Use O*Net OnLine to research a health care job
- Relate one's own experience to a specific health care opening during an interview

The *Instructor Resources* also contains visual aids that the instructor may display for classroom use, and handouts for student activities. There are activity visual aids that serve as formatting guides for the resume, reference list, cover letter, post-interview letter, reference letter, and resignation letter. These important aids will help the student perfect key health care industry documents. Several other visual aids offer useful information for classwork or future health care industry employment.

Additionally, *slides created in Microsoft PowerPoint*® are available for use in class lectures or as student handouts. Approximately 100 slides correspond to the steps in Sections 1 and 2 of the text.

The instructor resources are also available online and can be accessed via login.cengage.com or by contacting your sales representative.

## Also Available

BOOK ONLY: *How to Get a Job in Health Care,* 2nd Ed.
ISBN-13: 978-1-111-64010-1

StudyWARE™ with ResGen CD-ROM STANDALONE to accompany
*How to Get a Job in Health Care,* 2nd Ed. ISBN-13: 978-1-1116-4011-8

INSTANT ACCESS CODE for Premium Website to accompany
*How to Get a Job in Health Care,* 2nd Ed. ISBN-13: 978-1-133-60003-9

PRINTED ACCESS CARD for Premium Website to accompany
*How to Get a Job in Health Care,* 2nd Ed. ISBN-13: 978-1-133-60004-6

# About the Author

With over 40 years of instructional experience in business, work, and career education, Robert H. Zedlitz understands what is required for students to gain employment. His experience as an instructor and district coordinator in Work Experience Education in Fremont, California, gives him firsthand knowledge of the practical application of *How to Get a Job in Health Care*. His experience includes membership in the Fremont Unified School System District Curriculum Committee and the Career Education Consortium Committee for the California State Department of Education. He has a B.B.A. from the University of Toledo and an M.A. from the University of San Francisco. In addition to this text, he has authored *How to Get a Job Process Kit, 6th Ed.; Getting a Job Basic Process Kit; Getting a Job in the Travel Industry, 2nd Ed.;* and *The School to Work Planner, 3rd Ed.*

# Acknowledgments

The author is grateful for the Bureau of Labor Statistics information provided by O*Net OnLine, the *Occupational Outlook Handbook (OOH)*, and the Department of Labor's SCANS Report for America, 2000. These publications are a great reference for instructors and a benefit to job seekers. A special thanks must go to Matthew Seeley and Laura Wood of Cengage Learning, whose foresight made this second edition a reality. Thank you to the instructors who reviewed the manual and offered valuable suggestions. The reviewers include:

**Robin Douglas**

Medical Technology Instructor
Holmes Community College
Grenada, MS

**Celeste Fenton, Ph.D.**

Director of Faculty Professional
    Development at the Center for
    Innovative Teaching and Technology
    and Adjunct Professor for Career
    Decision Making
Hillsborough Community College
Tampa, Florida

**Donna A. Milner, BSN, RN**

Allied Health Instructor
Bucks County Technical High School
Fairless Hills, PA

**Christie Taylor, RN, BSN, MS Ed.**

Health Occupations Instructor, HOSA
    Advisor (Health Occupations
    Students of America)
Tyrone Area School District
Tyrone, Pennsylvania

# Introduction to Students

## Changes in Health Care

Health care is one of the largest and fastest-growing industries in the United States. According to the Bureau of Labor Statistics, 10 of the 20 occupations with the most job growth in 2012 and projected to 2020 are health related.[1]

The need for increased health care employment is in part the result of technological advances in patient care, an increased emphasis on preventive care, our aging population, and changes in public policy. Great advances have been made in medical knowledge. Americans today appreciate the benefits of preventing health problems. This attitude has helped develop a broad area of new services, health maintenance organizations, and employment opportunities. Modern medicine and health care awareness have enabled more people to live longer. The elderly make up a larger percentage of the population than ever before. Our aging population will create many changes and will open up new areas of the health care industry. Older people usually need more and different kinds of health care services than younger people.

Various health care reforms are now under consideration. These reforms may affect the number of people covered by some form of health insurance, the number of people being treated by health care providers, and the number and types of health care procedures that will be performed.

## Health Care Employment Opportunity

The health care and social assistance industry is projected to create about 28 percent of all new jobs created by the U.S. economy through the year 2020. This industry is expected to grow by 33 percent, or 5.7 million new jobs.[2] This presents a tremendous employment opportunity for trained men and women of every age and background. The health care industry offers many jobs that are challenging. Examples include the positions held by physicians, nurses, medical and dental assistants, technicians, technologists, or therapists. Health technicians and technologists work in occupations such as medical records and health information technicians, diagnostic medical sonographers, radiologic technologists and technicians, and dental hygienists. These workers may operate medical equipment and assist in diagnosing and treating patients. In addition, many health care workers are employed as support personnel performing clerical or maintenance tasks, or as workers in

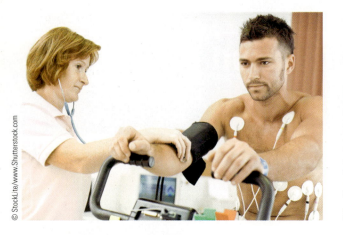
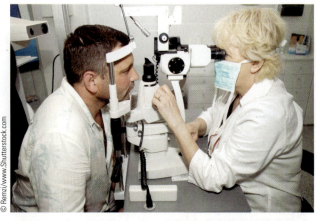
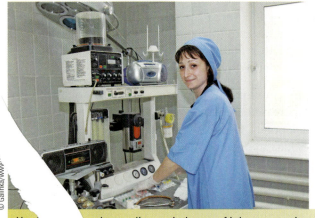
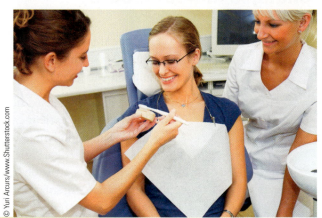

Health care is a large, diverse industry of job opportunity.

closely related industries. Examples include positions held by medical secretaries, transcriptionists, dieticians, nursing aides, orderlies, home health aides, and health care sales representatives.

# Technology Changes in Health Care

Different jobs are being created as the nature and scope of health care change and evolve. Technological advances have made many new procedures and methods of diagnosis and treatment possible. Technology in optics has improved with RetCam, a device that gives pediatric ophthalmologists a high-resolution photograph of an infant's eye allowing doctors to detect visual diseases that can lead to blindness and cancer. Clinical developments, such as infection control, less invasive surgical techniques, advances in reproductive technology, and gene therapy for cancer treatment, continue to increase the longevity and improve the quality of life of many Americans. Advances in medical technology also have improved the survival rates of trauma victims and the severely ill, who need extensive care from physical and occupational therapists and social workers as well as other support personnel.

In addition, advances in information technology have helped improve patient care and worker efficiency. Interpreters provide a vital link for non–English-speaking patients via video conference machines to translate between doctor and patient. Computers are used in almost all aspects of medical research, medical records, diagnostic testing, patient scheduling, and other health care provider services. Devices such as handheld computers are used to record a patient's medical history. Information on vital signs and orders for tests are transferred electronically to a main database. This process eliminates the need for paper and reduces record-keeping errors. Home health care has improved with remote monitoring of patients, video consultations, and long-distance nurse calls.

# What Health Care Job Do You Want?

Remember, you are not locked into any one particular job in the health care industry. It will be possible for you to make a job change with further training and education. You will certainly discover that a career in the health care industry affords you responsibility—and rewards you with advancement.

Whether you are getting your first job or contemplating an employment change, there are many interesting positions in the health care industry that can lead to a rewarding career. Many of the health care occupations projected to grow the fastest are among those listed here:

Clinical lab technician and
  technologist

Dental assistant

Dental hygienist

Dental lab technician

Dental secretary

Diagnostic medical sonographer

Diagnostic technician and technologist

Dietitian

Electrocardiograph technician

Emergency medical technician

Health information technician

Home health aide

Medical assistant

Medical biller/coder

Medical laboratory technician

Medical receptionist

Medical records technician

Medical secretary

Medical technologist

Medical transcriptionist

Nurse RN/LVN/LPN

Nursing assistant

Occupational therapy assistant

Ophthalmic medical assistant

Orthopedic therapy assistant

Paramedic

Pediatric assistant

Pharmacy technician

Physical therapy assistant

Physician assistant

Psychiatric assistant

Radiation therapy technologist

Radiologic technologist

Respiratory therapist

Surgical technologist

Veterinarian assistant

Vision care technician

X-ray technician

# A Tool for Your Success

The health care industry is rewarding. Health care occupations are growing twice as fast as the average occupations. As health care costs continue to rise, work is increasingly being delegated. For example, physician assistants, medical assistants, dental hygienists, and physical therapist aides are performing tasks that were previously performed by doctors, nurses, dentists, or other health care professionals. The move away from hospitalization also has created a significant increase nationwide in outpatient surgeries. Few industries offer such diverse employment opportunities. Many geographic areas, such as densely populated, inner-city areas and thinly populated, rural areas, are experiencing a shortage of health care workers. Due to the shortage of health care workers, and the need for employers to attract qualified health care workers, benefit programs are being improved. Opportunities such as tuition reimbursement, flex-time, and job-sharing are offered. To find the most rewarding job in health care, consider the many influences and changes in the field. Completing *How to Get a Job in Health Care* will add to your confidence in this challenge. This manual makes employment in the health care industry a reality, and leaving your job a positive career move.

## References

[1]*Employment Projections, Fastest Growing Occupations*, Bureau of Labor Statistics, U.S. Department of Labor, *Occupational Outlook Handbook*, 2012–13 Edition. http://bls.gov/emp/ep_table_103.htm

[2]*Healthcare and social assistance*, Bureau of Labor Statistics, U.S. Department of Labor, *Occupational Outlook Handbook*, 2012–13 Edition. http://www.bls.gov/ooh/about/projections-overview.htm

# Using This Text and StudyWARE™ with ResGen Software

## Understanding the Icons

Throughout this text, you will see these icons:

The **Activity Worksheets** icon indicates that there is a corresponding worksheet for an activity. The worksheets can be found in Section 3 of the text.

The **Portfolio Update** icon indicates when to add a document to your employment portfolio.

The **Website Icon** indicates when a website is used as part of an activity.

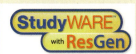

The **StudyWARE™ with ResGen** icon indicates when you should use the health care software for a fun quiz, game, photo, video, or to complete an employment planner, final resume, reference list, or letter.

## Using StudyWARE™ with ResGen

The StudyWARE™ with ResGen software includes the following items.

### Quizzes and Activities

Quizzes offer a helpful review of the major points discussed in each step. Quizzes include questions written in a variety of formats such as multiple choice, matching, and ordering/sorting, as well as a Hangman game for each step.

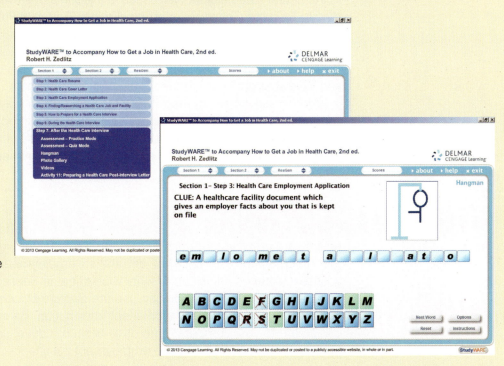

## Photo Gallery

The photo gallery is provided for you to view tips related to each step. Often a picture will trigger a reminder for you that will lead to success in your health care career.

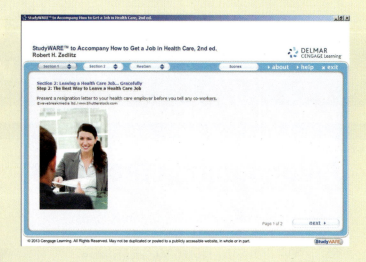

## Video Presentations

Throughout the software, videos are provided that demonstrate appropriate and inappropriate interview behavior. You will watch three job applicants go on interviews and hear from the interviewer and interviewee. Prompts in the text will alert you when to watch each video.

## Activity Worksheets in Electronic Format

All of the Activity Worksheets are provided in Microsoft® Word format on the software in order to facilitate electronic record-keeping.

## Resume Generator

Your software includes the Health Care Resume Generator. You will need an Internet connection in order to use the Resume Generator. This easy-to-use software will generate a variety of personalized resumes, a reference list, and employment letters designed specifically to help you find a rewarding job in the health care field, as well as leave a job in a positive manner. If you are new to Resume Generator, start by clicking "Edit Your Profile" to enter your personal resume information. Your Profile stores your personal information so your Resume Generator can create new employment documents for you in the future. IMPORTANT: Before exiting Resume Generator, you must export and save your profile information to your computer hard drive or thumb drive in order to use it again in the future. Returning users may then upload the previously saved profile information using the "Upload Your Profile" button in the Resume Generator. Always save any generated files to your computer hard drive or thumb drive, and place a copy in your employment portfolio for future employment assistance.

### Sample Documents

The *Sample Documents* in your software give you an additional way to create health care employment documents. The *Sample Documents* include the same four resumes, the reference list, and the six employment letters as shown in your text. After you finish an Activity Worksheet in Section 3 of your text to draft one of these documents, you can use the *Sample Document* in your software and edit it with your activity worksheet information. Be sure to save the files you create to your computer hard drive or thumb drive, and place a copy in your employment portfolio for future employment assistance.

## Supporting Documents

Your software also contains seven *Supporting Documents* that you may use to plan and supplement *How to Get a Job in Health Care* activities. The *Supporting Documents* include all the planner files listed in the chart.

## Sample and Supporting Electronic Files Chart

The chart shown here gives the title and file name, corresponding section and step number, and specific directions for each of the files listed.

| Section 1 | Title and *File Name* | Directions |
|---|---|---|
| **Step** | | |
| 1 | Standard Resume<br>*Sample_Resume-Standard.doc*<br>Chronological Resume<br>*Sample_Resume-Chronological.doc*<br>Functional Resume<br>*Sample_Resume-Functional.doc*<br>Combination Resume<br>*Sample_Resume-Combination.doc* | Four health care resume formats appear on your computer screen. Select and edit the health care resume that is appropriate for you. Use your corresponding resume activity practice sheet for editing information. DO NOT EDIT RESUME HEADINGS. Supply your personal information under each heading. Maintain suggested resume spacing when editing your resume. |
| 1 | Reference List<br>*Sample_ReferenceList.doc* | A reference list format appears on your computer screen. Edit this reference list, keeping the main heading and using the suggested spacing. |
| 2 | Cover Letter Planner<br>*CoverLetterPlanner.doc* | Before keying your health care cover letter, use this planner to outline your main cover letter points. Keep in mind that the primary objective of a cover letter is to secure an interview. |
| 2 | Cover Letter 1<br>*Sample_CoverLetter1.doc*<br>Cover Letter 2<br>*Sample_CoverLetter2.doc*<br>Cover Letter 3<br>*Sample_CoverLetter3.doc* | Three health care cover letter formats appear on your computer screen. Select and edit the health care cover letter that is appropriate for you. Use information from your software cover letter planner and corresponding Section 3 cover letter activity practice sheet for editing. Maintain suggested spacing when editing your cover letter. |

(*continues*)

| Section 1 | Title and *File Name* | Directions |
|---|---|---|
| **Step** | | |
| 4 | Job Search Planner<br><br>*JobSearchPlanner.doc* | A successful health care job search requires organization and effort. The weekly planner allows you to set goals for generating a number of health care job leads, setting up a specific number of interviews, or making contact with a specific health care facility. |
| 5, 6, 7 | Interview Planner<br><br>*InterviewPlanner.doc* | During an extensive job search you may find it difficult to remember details of every meeting. That is why it is important to develop a record-keeping system for all your interviews. This planner records details, reminders, notes, and contacts. |
| 7 | Post-Interview Letter Planner<br><br>*PostInterviewLetterPlanner.doc* | Before writing your post-interview letter, you may find it helpful to determine your key points. This planner helps you identify what is important to say in your post-interview letter. |
| 7 | Post-Interview Letter<br><br>*Sample_PostInterviewLetter.doc* | A sample post-interview letter appears on your computer screen. Edit this letter using information from your software post-interview letter planner and your Section 3 practice activity sheet. Maintain suggested spacing when editing your post-interview letter. |
| 7 | Job Offer Evaluator<br><br>*JobOfferEvaluator.doc* | The decision to accept or reject a health care job offer is an important one. This job offer evaluator helps you make a decision about one job or helps you compare several offers. |

| Section 2 | Title and *File Name* | Directions |
|---|---|---|
| **Step** | | |
| 2 | Exit Conversation and Resignation Letter Planner<br><br>*ExitConversationandResignation LetterPlanner.doc* | Before writing a resignation letter or having an exit conversation with your employer, good planning will ensure your leaving is positive. This planner helps you organize your thoughts. |
| 2 | Resignation Letter<br><br>*Sample_ResignationLetter.doc* | A sample resignation letter appears on your computer screen. Edit this letter using information from your software resignation letter planner and your Section 3 resignation letter practice activity sheet. Maintain suggested spacing when editing your resignation letter. |
| 3 | Reference Letter Planner<br><br>*ReferenceLetterPlanner.doc* | When you are given permission to draft a letter of reference about yourself for someone else's signature, put yourself in that person's shoes. This planner will help you outline how someone sees you. |
| 3 | Reference Letter<br><br>*Sample_ReferenceLetter.doc* | A sample health care reference letter appears on your computer screen. Edit this letter using information from your software reference letter planner and your Section 3 reference letter practice activity. |

# Getting and Starting a Job in Health Care

## Introduction

Almost everyone needs to polish basic job-hunting skills. This employment guide, *How to Get a Job in Health Care,* offers students, the recent graduate, or person who plans to enter or return to the workforce an easy-to-follow, step-by-step guide for obtaining and starting a career position in the health care industry.

The eight steps in Section 1, Getting and Starting a Job in Health Care, follow, along with a summary of what each step includes.

### Step 1: Health Care Resume

This step contains many important questions about resumes and carefully explains how to develop a resume. Four sample resumes and a reference list are included, with detailed guidelines to ensure that the resumes you construct are effective.

### Step 2: Health Care Cover Letter

This step deals with the cover letter and its importance in looking for a health care job. Three sample cover letters and instructions tell what a cover letter should say and how to write one.

### Step 3: Health Care Employment Application

This step deals with what health care employers look for in employment applications. A sample employment application and two practice application forms are included. You will learn the necessary information and materials you need to successfully complete your employment applications.

### Step 4: Finding and Researching a Health Care Job and Facility

This step outlines the most important sources of health care job leads and how to pursue them. You will research a health care job and health care facility that may have the job you want, and develop your network of people who can help you get a job interview. You will learn how a business card and a thank-you note will give you an edge for a health care job opening.

### Step 5: How to Prepare for a Health Care Interview

This step tells what information to take to a health care job interview and how to appear your best. You will learn why researching the health care facility and the job description is important before a health care job interview. Included are 12 of the most common interview questions and suggested answers.

### Step 6: During the Health Care Interview

This step explains what to do during an interview and how to contact the health care employer for a hiring decision. A model health care interview, interview case study activity, and a "Do's and Don'ts" checklist are included.

### Step 7: After the Health Care Interview

This step outlines what to do after a health care interview to give you an edge over your competitors. You will learn how to write a successful post-interview letter and a thank-you note, as well as what to say in a phone call and an e-mail, to follow up for a health care hiring decision.

### Step 8: How to Start a Health Care Job

This section ends with advice for making a professional first impression when you start your new health care job. You will learn how to talk to your supervisor so you can "ace" your performance review. After all of your hard work getting your dream job, these suggestions will give you confidence to gain the trust of your new health care co-workers and supervisor.

# Health Care Resume

## In this step you will find

- the definition of resume.

- reasons why your health care resume is important.

- instructions for writing your health care resume.

- an activity checklist of employment power words and phrases.

- an activity to write health care job objectives.

- four sample health care resumes and writing activities.

- an activity to construct a health care reference list.

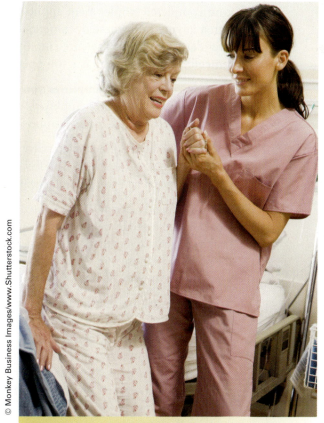

Make sure your resume draws a clear connection between your skills and the health care job opening.

## What Is a Resume?

A resume is a personal data sheet. It is a short summary of important facts about you. These facts help a health care employer decide whether or not you are an appropriate candidate for health care jobs. Any person who is serious about seeking a job in the health care field should always have a well-thought-out, up-to-date, and well-prepared resume.

# Why Is Your Health Care Resume Important?

The purpose of a resume is to get an interview. Remember, the resume is the health care employer's first look at you. An effective resume may make the potential health care employer want to know more about you. It must be accurate and error free so you make a good first impression.

You should prepare a health care resume for the following reasons.

- **To help you complete a health care employment application quickly and accurately.** An employment application is a form used by many medical organizations to gather information about a job candidate. Employment applications are discussed in detail in Step 3.

- **To demonstrate your potential as a health care worker.** Resumes provide additional information and reflect a health care job applicant's potential better than an employment application. When you visit a health care employer at a job fair or a job site, give the employer a copy of your resume along with your completed employment application, even if you do not have an interview. Often having both these documents on file will help you get an interview at a later date. Once a health care employer has met you face-to-face, you may be remembered when there is a job opening.

- **To show a health care employer you are organized, prepared, and serious about getting a job.** Health care employers often consider you an above-average candidate for a job because your resume is well-written and accurate.

- **To feel self-assured during an interview because important facts and dates are in front of you.** Having a resume helps you feel prepared and professional and adds to your self-confidence when you present a health care employer your reasons to be hired.

- **To mail, or send electronically to potential health care employers with whom you would like to arrange an interview.** You can send copies of your resume to more health care employers than you can visit. This saves you time and money. Remember, the primary purpose of a health care resume is to convince someone to interview you for a health care job. Be sure to include a cover letter with any resume you send.

You may want to fax or e-mail your resume, or post it on health care employer websites or online job sites. Health care employers' career center websites usually give directions for submitting your electronic resume. Be aware, however, that electronic resumes have a different format than traditional resumes. You can convert your MS Word resumes to plain text, e-mail, and scannable versions and save them on your thumb drive ready to submit to various online health care job sites. To see how to create electronic resumes, ready to copy and paste online, or into your e-mail message, go to www.susanireland.com.

Be sure to protect your privacy and create a separate, professional e-mail address to use on your resume instead of your personal e-mail address. You might use your first name initial and your last name, such as jstanley@gmail.com. The following sites offer free e-mail accounts: Hotmail.com, Gmail.com, and Yahoo.com.

**WEBSITE**

- **To distribute to relatives, friends, guidance counselors, teachers, character references, and other persons who are willing to help you find a health care job.** Your resume gives these important people in your network a clear picture of your qualifications. It also acts as a constant reminder that you are seeking health care employment. A health care job lead could very well result from one of these close contacts.

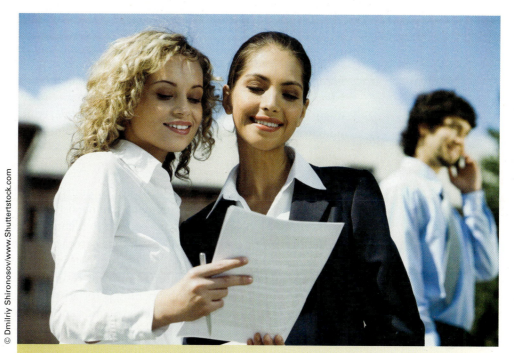

© Dmitriy Shironosov/www.Shutterstock.com

Distribute your resume to your network of people who are willing to help you find a health care job.

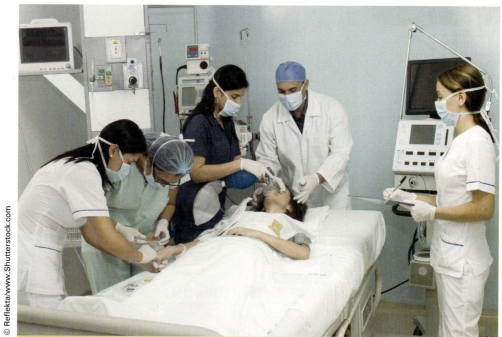

© Reflekta/www.Shutterstock.com

Consider your clinical internship when you write your resume.

# What Should Be Included on a Resume?

Resumes are written in many different styles. Four resume styles are included here: standard, chronological, functional, and combination. However, there are basic elements that most often are included in any resume style. These basic elements include personal information, job objective, education, work experience, qualifications for the job position, and a statement that references are available.

## Job Objective

Notice that each of the sample resumes contains a job objective. At this time in your health care academic experience you most likely have a job objective. You can write a job objective on your resume to identify a specific health care job title, type of health care work, or a health care career goal. Then the contents of your resume can be tailored to your job objective. If you know of a specific health care job opening, include a job objective on your resume specific to that opening. For example, if the health care job opening is for a psychiatric aide, your job objective could say: "To work as a psychiatric aide specializing in helping children who have autism." Here are other examples of job objectives:

- To work as a nurse (LVN) in a recognized health care environment.

- To obtain a dental laboratory assistant position.

- To work as an EKG technician for a hospital.

- To work as an entry-level surgical technologist in a hospital.

- To join a private practice as a physician's medical assistant.

If you are exploring the health care job field, and have not made a definite job choice, you may not want your resume to state a job objective. The advantage is that the prospective employer may consider you for more than one job opening. The disadvantage is that a prospective employer may not want to take the time to analyze your resume to decide for which job you are best qualified.

Carefully read Figure 1.1.1, Guidelines for Creating a Standard Health Care Resume, and the A–H descriptions of each section. See how each description compares to the same A–H sections of the standard style resume, Figure 1.1.2.

Now examine the remaining three resume styles. Figure 1.1.3 is a chronological resume, Figure 1.1.4 is a functional resume, and Figure 1.1.5 is a combination resume. Notice they are written in different styles, but all contain the same basic elements of successful resumes.

# What Resume Style Is Best for You?

Good judgment is necessary to determine which health care resume would be the most effective for getting you an interview. Study the descriptions of the four resume samples and decide which style best describes your work experience and skills.

- **Standard resume:** Look at Figure 1.1.2, the sample standard resume. Notice the standard resume information is organized by category. This makes the standard resume easy to develop. You can quickly fill in the blanks under each heading.

It clearly shows a prospective health care employer your personal information, job objective, education, and your work experience with responsibilities, duties, and work skills. A standard resume can also emphasize memberships, honors, and special skills. Everyone has special skills that are transferable to a variety of health care jobs. Think of skills that you have acquired through hobbies, volunteering, and any activity or life experience. Teamwork, writing, time management, and effective listening are examples of skills used in most health care jobs. First-time job seekers and recent graduates might feel more comfortable developing a standard resume.

- **Chronological resume:** Look at Figure 1.1.3, the sample chronological resume.

  At the top of your chronological resume, place your health care job objective, followed by a description of your job objective qualifications, including your education.

  Notice the chronological resume lists work experiences in order of time. Your work experience is dated with the most recent experience listed first. Use this style to show steady employment without gaps or a great number of job changes.

- **Functional resume:** Look at Figure 1.1.4, the sample functional resume. The functional resume highlights what you know, what you have accomplished, and what you have achieved through your education. Notice that the functional resume is a series of skill clusters that identify a job candidate's most important qualifications. You can arrange your experience around responsibilities related to your health care job objective. List your most important work experience first. You may also want to use this format when you have gaps in employment and/or lack experience directly related to your health care job objective.

- **Combination resume:** Look at Figure 1.1.5, the sample combination resume. Notice the combination resume combines chronological and functional resume styles. It gives the work experience directly related to the health care job opening by most recent date first and arranges the resume information in skill clusters. Specific job skills are listed to capture the employers' attention for a match with the position requirements. Use this format if you have limited experience or want to highlight your accomplishments directed to a particular health care job opening.

## Creating Your Perfect Health Care Resume

To create a professional-looking health care resume, study the sample resumes. Notice the margin and spacing guidelines. Refer to the Formatting Guidelines, which explain how to format your resume. Your resume will be organized and readable if you include section headings and add space between sections. Keep in mind, though, a one-page resume is preferred.

**FIGURE 1.1.1** Standard Resume Descriptions for Figure 1.1.2

## Guidelines for Creating a
## Standard Health Care Resume

**Ⓐ PERSONAL INFORMATION**

List your name, address, telephone and cell number, and e-mail address. The prospective health care employer may need to know some additional facts about you, but this information must stay within the bounds of your state's fair employment laws. The prospective employer will use this information to contact you.

**Ⓑ JOB OBJECTIVE**

The job objective states the health care position you are seeking. It should be a clearly and concisely written sentence of your job goal. For example: "To work as a licensed Vocational Nurse at a well-managed convalescent hospital." A well-written job objective can also include a career goal or the ultimate job position you would like to achieve in the health care field. Your job objective and career goal should be closely related. For exa    "To work for a large hospital as a Medical Record Technician, which could lead to a position as      .cal Record Supervisor."

**Ⓒ EDUCATION**

List the schoo'          ave attended in reverse chronological order (most recent first). Include dates of attendan                 .e and location of the schools, the curriculum studied (general education, medical                    .ssisting, college preparatory, etc.), and the degree, diploma, certificate, or license                  .ny courses that relate to your career objective. High school records may or may not be                are still attending school, place your expected graduation month and year in parentheses            your diploma or degree. For example: Licensed Vocational Nurse Certificate (June, 20—).

**Ⓓ WORK EXPERIENCE**

List all full-time, part-time, summer, or volunteer jobs. Be sure to list any internship. Present your work experience in reverse chronological order (most recent first). Include dates of employment, names and locations of the health care facilities or organizations, job titles, work responsibilities, and duties. Show how your previous work and skills apply to your job objective and career goal.

**Ⓔ MEMBERSHIPS**

Include memberships in professional health care organizations or other career-related clubs and associations. This shows that you are willing to donate valuable time to worthy causes without compensation. Use good judgment, however, before listing religious, political, or any other sensitive organization memberships. You may not want to disclose any memberships that are not job related. If you have no memberships, eliminate this section.

**Ⓕ HONORS**

List any honors, special certificates of achievement, and awards you have received. If you had a high class ranking, record it here. If you have no honors or special awards, eliminate this section.

**Ⓖ SPECIAL SKILLS**

List any special skills that you wish to highlight even if they are not job related. A prospective employer should be aware of all your talents. For example: Microsoft Exel, and speaking knowledge of Spanish. If you have no special skills, eliminate this section. Remember, however, skills such as communication, flexibility, and organization are skills that will transfer to many health care jobs.

**Ⓗ REFERENCES**

Place the following statement at the bottom of your resume: "References available." Key and provide a separate list of references when you interview. The name, business title (if any), company or organization, address, and telephone number of your references are usually required. Be sure to ask permission of those references you plan to provide. Include former employers, instructors, doctors, nurses, or friends well established in business or the health care field who know your character and accomplishments and will speak well of you. See Figure 1.1.6 for an example of a reference list.

1″ (Line 7)

**(A)** **PERSONAL INFORMATION**            **SARAH PEREZ**
8425 Lincoln Lane, Bowling Green, OH 43403
(419) 555-1258 Cell (419) 555-8686
sperez@gmail.com
2–4S

**(B)** **JOB OBJECTIVE**            To obtain a position as a Dental Assistant
2S

**(C)** **EDUCATION**            2S
20-- to 20--            Toledo Medical-Dental College
Toledo, OH
Program: Dental Assisting
Dental Assistant Certification, June, 20--.
2S

20-- to 20--            Woodward High School
Toledo, OH
Degree: High School Diploma
2S

> To prepare a professional looking resume, follow the formatting guides shown. Remember **2S** means double space (or two returns), **4S** means quadruple space (four returns). Do not include this information on your resume.

1″                                                                      1″

**(D)** **WORK EXPERIENCE**
20-- to present            Brent J. Lin, D.D.S.
450 Temple Court
Toledo, OH
Dental Assistant---Internship
Responsibilities/Duties: General office procedures including appointments, dental bookkeeping, collections, and insurance forms. Dental assisting duties including X-rays, plaque control therapy, dental radiography, nutrition and preventive dentistry, tray set-ups, chair side assisting, laboratory and sterilization procedures.
2S

20-- to 20--            North American Alarm Co.
4515 Howard Street
Bowling Green, OH
Dispatcher
Responsibilities/Duties: Dispatch service alarm calls, handle phone communication, and develop customer leads.
2S

**(E)** **MEMBERSHIPS**            American Dental Assistants Association
Bowling Green Photography Club
2S

**(F)** **HONORS**            Certificate of Academic Achievement, class rank fifth, Toledo Medical-Dental College.
2S

**(G)** **SPECIAL SKILLS**            Windows XP, Microsoft Word, Excel, keying 80 WPM, Spanish language proficient
2S

**(H)** **REFERENCES**            References available.

**FIGURE 1.1.3** Chronological Resume

1″ (Line 7)

**LISA BROWN**
8312 Broadway
Arlington Heights, IL 60004
(847) 555-4732
Cell (847) 555-3197
lbrown@yahoo.com

*JOB OBJECTIVE*        2S

To join a leading health clinic as a Medical Records Technician. Future goal
is to manage a medical facility.
        2S

*QUALIFICATIONS*

        2S
Clinical Experience: 20--
- Recognized for considerate patient intake.
- Strong listening skills assisting patients, coordinated with staff to create smooth relations.
- Most proud of supervisor commendation for transcribing accurate medical reports.
- Quickly learned to process insurance forms.
- Proficient in Microsoft Access, IDX Systems, Visionary Medical Systems, Visionary Office PM, QM Software Receivables Management.
        2S
Education: Chicago Community College, A.A. Degree,
Medical Records Technician, June, 20--.
Registered Health Information Technician, (RHIT), 20--.
        2S

*EMPLOYERS*

        2S
May, 20-- to Jun 20--        Memorial Hospital
Chicago, IL
Directed Internship
        2S
May, 20-- to Present        Midland Trust Company
Chicago, IL
Merchant Teller
        2S
Apr, 20-- to Mar, 20--        Payless Shoes
Chicago, IL
Salesperson
        2S

*REFERENCES*        References available.

1″        1″

**FIGURE 1.1.6** Reference List

1 1/2″ or 2″ (Line 10 or 13)

**REFERENCES OF SARAH PEREZ**
8425 Lincoln Lane, Bowling Green, OH 43403
(419) 555-1258 Cell (419) 555-8686
sperez@gmail.com

4S

Brent Lin, D.D.S.
450 Temple Court
Toledo, OH 43604
(419) 555-3131

4S

Naomi Mesky, D.D.S. (instructor)
Toledo Dental College
8554 Canyon Avenue
Toledo, OH 43604
(419) 555-4165

2″

5S

William Landry, Manager
North American Alarm Company
4515 Howard Street
Bowling Green, OH 43403
(419) 555-6230

4S

Howard Smith
Bowling Green Community Bank
6161 Main Street
Bowling Green, OH 43403
(419) 555-4672

### In this step you will find

- the definition of a health care cover letter.
- guidelines for writing a health care cover letter.
- three sample health care cover letters.
- a health care cover letter writing activity.

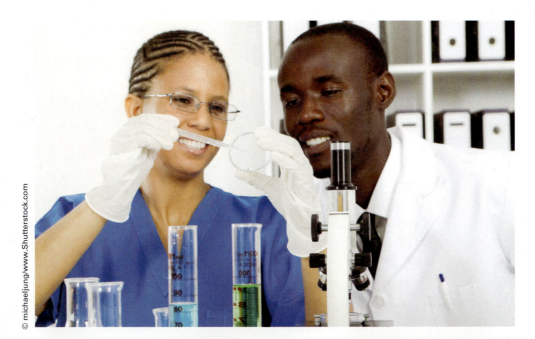

© michaeljung/www.Shutterstock.com

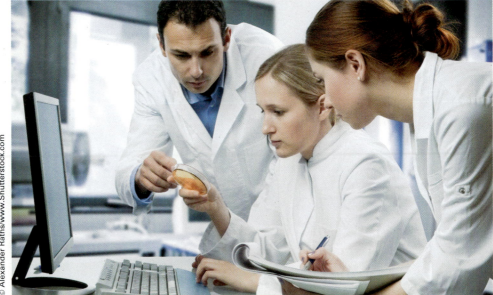

© Alexander Raths/www.Shutterstock.com

Skills learned in school such as teamwork and research are important to many health care employers.

# What Is a Health Care Cover Letter?

A cover letter is your personal introduction that states the job for which you are applying, your qualifications, and your request for an interview. Your cover letter is important as it may be the first contact you have with a prospective health care employer. Remember the rewards of a good first impression. Always use a cover letter whenever you send a resume to a prospective health care employer, or present your resume in person.

# How Should You Write a Health Care Cover Letter?

Use the following guidelines when writing a health care cover letter:

1. Address your letter to a specific person, if possible. If you do not have the name of the contact person, call the health care facility and ask for the name of the human resource manager or the supervisor in the service area in which you want to work. Some medical employment ads do not contain the name of a contact person, medical organization name, or street and city address; instead, a fax number or P.O. box replaces an address. See the sample cover letter, Figure 1.2.1, to see where to place a fax number.

   If you cannot obtain an individual's name, create a greeting by adding the word "manager" to the hiring department—for example, *Dear Human Resource Manager*, or *Dear Human Relations Manager, or Dear Personnel Manager*. You can also add the word "manager" to the service area that has the position you want. Or you can add the word "manager" to the job title you want—for example, *Dear Medical Office Manager*, or *Dear Dental Office Receptionist Manager*, or *Dear Vocational Nurse Manager*. Read the sample cover letter, Figure 1.2.1, to see how a greeting was created.

2. State the purpose of your letter and the health care position for which you are applying.

3. State those qualifications that make you well suited for the health care position.

4. Request an interview.

5. Sign your letter before sending it.

Your health care cover letter paragraphs should be brief, clear, and carefully written. Proofread your letter for content and spelling. Have someone who is proficient in grammar edit your letter for correct spelling, punctuation, and grammar. **Remember, any error in your cover letter will reflect poorly on you.** Be sure to include a copy of your resume with each cover letter. Also include any other requested information, such as samples of your work.

## Content of a Health Care Cover Letter

The content of a cover letter varies considerably depending upon the health care position you are seeking. Your health care cover letter paragraphs should include the following:

1. **Opening paragraph.** State why you are writing, the name of the health care position for which you are applying, and how you learned of the opening. If you are responding to an ad, state the date and name of the newspaper or other source in which you saw the ad.

**FIGURE 1.2.1** Cover Letter

1" (Line 7)

**SOPHIA DAVIS**

2280 Walnut Drive, Chicago, IL 60610 - (312) 555-0184 - Cell (312) 555-7219

sd@aol.com

2-4S

> **MEDICAL OFFICE ASSISTANT**
>
> Fast paced valley clinic. Org. & multi-task skills. Excellent benefits. Fax resume to (312) 555-0168.

1"

April 15, 20--

4S

1"

Fax No. (312) 555-0168

2S

Dear Medical Office Manager

2S

**A** After all of my training, I am motivated to begin my career in health care. The Medical Office Assistant position, for which I am applying, was advertised in the April 13th Chicago Tribune.

2S

My clinical training gave me the skills to assist a physician and other medical personnel. I look forward to using the administrative and computer skills I learned in my medical office training. The medical coding and billing systems I used have prepared me for this job. I am most proud of my ability to schedule and receive patients and understand their needs. I have a passion for helping patients with their medical problems.

2S

**B** Personal Skills:
- Positive work attitude benefits medical team and patients.
- Experienced working with various medical insurance forms.
- Understand and appreciate confidentiality and patient rights.
- Diversity experienced.
- Excellent track record organizing for productivity.

2S

**C** I will follow-up this week for a time that you can meet with me to discuss my resume and how I can contribute to your medical office team.

2S

Sincerely

*Sophia Davis*    4S

Sophia Davis

2S

Enclosure

> To prepare a professional looking letter, follow the formatting guides shown. Remember **2S** means double space (or two returns), **4S** means quadruple space (four returns). Do not include this information on your cover letter.
>
> **A** Purpose of letter
>
> **B** Qualifications or reasons why applicant should be interviewed
>
> **C** Request for an interview

2. **Middle paragraph.** State why you are interested in working for the medical organization and why you desire this type of work. This is a good place to bring attention to your personal qualities and work skills. Point out your special qualifications, achievements, and training.

3. **Closing paragraph.** Refer to your resume and encourage action. Ask for an interview or end with a question that encourages a reply. Instead of a statement such as "I would appreciate hearing from you in the future," which does not draw action, you might say, "I will call you next week to determine when we might meet to discuss the health care job opening." Or you may say, "Please call me at (837) 555-0154 concerning an interview to discuss this health care opening."

## Sample Cover Letters

Two sample ads and the health care cover letters that were written in response to them are presented in this step. In the first cover letter, Figure 1.2.1, Sophia Davis is applying for her first health care position as a medical office assistant. Shinae Cho, a recent graduate, writes the second health care cover letter, Figure 1.2.2. She is responding to a medical employment ad for a nurse's aide position. The third health care cover letter, Figure 1.2.3, shows that Thomas Lewis has followed up a contact from Mrs. Mayo, the placement officer for Hayward Dental Assisting College, concerning a job lead. He is sending a resume and cover letter to Ms. Toshi Yukimura.

Read the health care employment ads, Figure 1.2.4, and notice that none of them ask for a cover letter. However, employers recognize that a cover letter shows a job applicant's extra effort and Sophia, Shinae, and Thomas all want jobs! The ad Sophia is responding to uses a fax number instead of a name or address. Sophia had two choices: she could send a cover letter without a greeting or add the title "Manager" to the medical office that has the job for which she is applying. She chose the latter. Shinae sends her cover letter and resume to the person identified in the ad, and Thomas sends his cover letter and resume to the person to whom his placement officer referred him. Make sure you follow the directions in the ad exactly or your cover letter and resume may be disregarded.

Notice that all three job candidates state the purpose of their letter, list their medical job qualifications or reasons why they should be interviewed for the position, and request an interview. Also notice that the candidates include their telephone number, cell phone number, and e-mail address. Try to make it as convenient as possible for an employer to reach you to establish a time for an interview.

Sophia uses her cover letter to explain how her clinical training and medical office training qualify her for the job. Remember, even if you have little or no paid or volunteer work experience, you can still use your school courses, training, including internship experience, relevant skills, strong personal qualities, and interests to develop a winning cover letter.

Some health care employers may request that you use their website or mobile site to respond to a job opening. Health care employer websites may request that you first complete an online job information form before submitting your resume and cover letter.

**FIGURE 1.2.2** Cover Letter

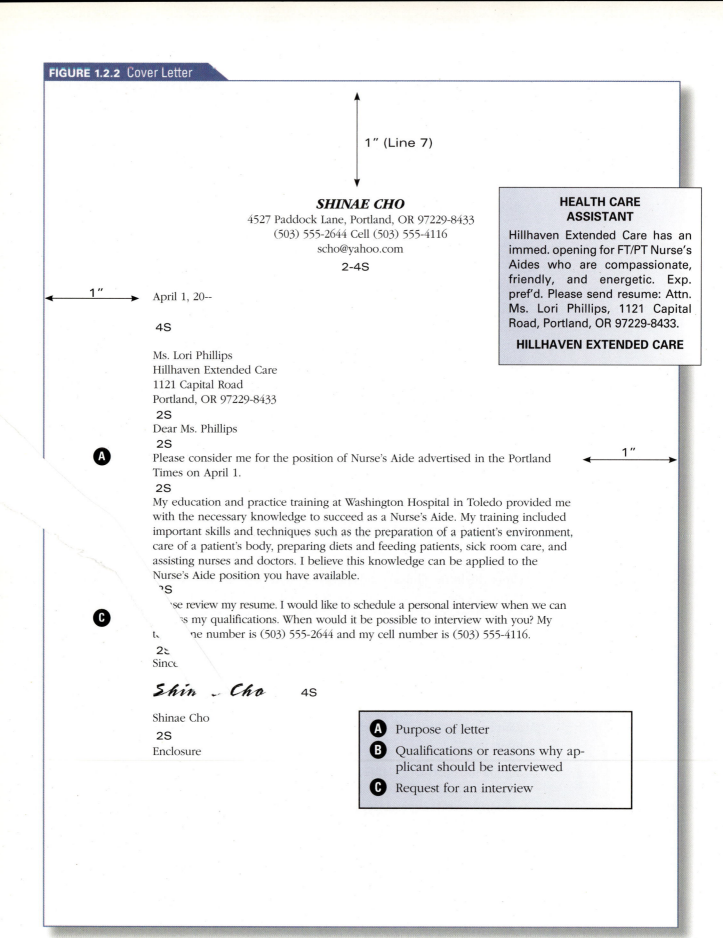

1" (Line 7)

**SHINAE CHO**
4527 Paddock Lane, Portland, OR 97229-8433
(503) 555-2644 Cell (503) 555-4116
scho@yahoo.com

2-4S

1"

April 1, 20--

4S

Ms. Lori Phillips
Hillhaven Extended Care
1121 Capital Road
Portland, OR 97229-8433

2S

Dear Ms. Phillips

2S

**Ⓐ** Please consider me for the position of Nurse's Aide advertised in the Portland Times on April 1.

2S

My education and practice training at Washington Hospital in Toledo provided me with the necessary knowledge to succeed as a Nurse's Aide. My training included important skills and techniques such as the preparation of a patient's environment, care of a patient's body, preparing diets and feeding patients, sick room care, and assisting nurses and doctors. I believe this knowledge can be applied to the Nurse's Aide position you have available.

?S

**Ⓒ** se review my resume. I would like to schedule a personal interview when we can s my qualifications. When would it be possible to interview with you? My t ne number is (503) 555-2644 and my cell number is (503) 555-4116.

2S

Since

*Shin  Cho*     4S

Shinae Cho

2S

Enclosure

**Ⓐ** Purpose of letter

**Ⓑ** Qualifications or reasons why applicant should be interviewed

**Ⓒ** Request for an interview

**FIGURE 1.2.3** Cover Letter

1″ (Line 7)

**THOMAS LEWIS**
2600 Lambert Ave., Skokie, IL 60174
(217) 555-4411
Cell (217) 555-2719
tlewis@gmail.com
2-4S

1″

March 1, 20--

4S

Ms. Toshi Yukimura, Office Manager
Paul Mercado, D.D.S., Inc.
3420 Ridge Lane
Springfield, IL 62702

2S

Dear Ms. Yukimura

2S

1″

**A** Mrs. Mayo, placement officer for Hayward Dental Assisting College, has advised me of a Dental Assistant opening with your office. Please consider me an applicant for this position.

2S

**B** I will graduate from Hayward Dental Assisting College in June, with a certificate in Dental Assisting. My school training and field internship have provided me with the professional skills to succeed as a qualified Dental Assistant. Training included office necessary management procedures, patient relations, and clinical procedures such as chair side assisting. These skills and other acquired dental assisting training would make me a valuable employee in the position you have open.

2S

**C** Please review the enclosed resume. I would appreciate an interview to discuss my background and will call March 7 for an appointment.

2S

Sincerely

*Thomas Lewis*    4S

Thomas Lewis

2S

Enclosure

**A** Purpose of letter
**B** Qualifications or reasons why applicant should be interviewed
**C** Request for an interview

**FIGURE 1.2.4** Newspaper Employment Ads

## MEDICAL TECHNOLOGIST

New Pathology Institute has immediate opening for P/T Med. Tech with Toxicology background, Nights (11 P.M.-7 A.M.), Thur., Fri., Sat. Great benefits. Minimum 1 year experience. Florida Clinical Toxicologist license or MT (ASCP) required. Ability to troubleshoot.

F/T, P/T, or on-call openings also exist in the following categories:

MED TECH - Hematology, Blood Bank Chemistry, Coagulation, Urinalysis, Toxicology, and Microbiology.

Other positions are available in areas of SPECIMEN PROCESSING, LABORATORY ASSISTING, COURIER, PHLEBOTOMY, and LAB OFFICE (CLERICAL).

For immediate consideration, forward cover letter, stating area of interest, and resume to Beverly Martin, New Pathology Institute, 2920 Telegraph Ave., Miami, FL 33134.

**PEDIATRIC** Dentist Children's Dental Center, a busy, heavily restorative practice seeks full-time pediatric dentists for locations in San Jose and Sunnyvale. Multiple openings. Two years experience with high-risk patients Send resumes to Anastasia at P.O. Box 425 Monterey, CA 93905.

**MEDICAL** ASSISTANT Part time, back office in ObGyn practice. Spanish helpful. Compensation depends on experience. Fax resume to 510 555 7107.

### MEDICAL NP/PA

Very busy MD in Concord seeking lic. NP or PA to join our fast paced family/occ.med.practice immed. Pay $55/hr. w/full bnfts. Call Millie 465-555-6140. Fax res. 465-555-7635.

### MEDICAL BILLER

**Premier Physical Therapy & Wellness,** is seeking qualified candidates for a **Medical Billing position**. Positions are generally full time. Experience is required. Please attach an updated resume when applying for this position. MUST have the skills and qualifications with 2+ years of combined experience as a physical therapy / rehabilitation medical biller including collections. Interested candidate should senders to Ann Evans 3224 Hill Ave Ft. Worth, TX 76103.

## HEALTHCARE

**PATIENT ADVOCATE** Growing healthcare office seeks analytical prof. w/detail knowledge of MEDICAL rules & regulations. Must be detail oriented & have excel. verbal/written communication skills. Must be computer lit. Bilingual Spanish. San Jose & /or San Mateo area. Fax res. 650-555-2549.

### MEDICAL FRONT OFFICE RECEPTIONIST

For busy Surgery Office. Must be able to work independently & be detail oriented w/excellent org., communication & multitask skills. Competitive salary & excellent benefits. Fax resume 510-555-6822.

NEW
PATHOLOGY
INSTITUTE

MEDICAL-HOME CARE

### RESPIRATORY TECH.

If you value personal independence on the job, if you care about really making a positive contribution to the lives of people needing home medical care, if you are serious about building a CAREER, with ADVANCEMENT POTENTIAL in the home health industry, Americair wants you.

Americair is Ft. Worth's fastest growing home health care company seeking to expand our family-like technical staff by adding several FULL TIME home care medical technicians.

This territory based career opportunity offers a complete TRAINING program, full BENEFITS and a competitive SALARY RANGE.

Applicants need to send resume: Stephanie Manor, 846 Malibar Rd., Ft. Worth, TX 76116, or Fax (817) 555-2151.

### ★ ★ DENTAL ★ ★ ★ ★ ASSISTANT ★ ★

F/T. Come join our team. Ultra modern office & growing practice has opening for quality-oriented person. X-RAY LIC. NEEDED.

Send resume: James Black, D.D.S. 301 Main Street, Louisville, KY 40206.

## PHYSICAL THERAPIST

Boothington Medical Offices in Fairfield is seeking a licensed Physical Therapist with outpatient orthopedic experience for a one year (half-time) position. You will also function as a case manager in special projects for patients with low back pain. Send resume to: Ray Vasquez, M.D., 2201 Phillips Ave., Fairfield, CA 94533. We are an EEO/AA employer. Minorities, women, handicapped and veterans are encouraged to apply.

**BOOTHINGTON**
Always There Always Caring

### MEDICAL CLAIMS COLLECTOR/CODER

Exper. necessary. F/T position. Familiarity with RVS, CPT-4 & ICD-9 codes. Send resume: Mr. Segio Caro, 1313 Montez Rd., San Antonio, TX 78234.

**Physical Therapist Asst.**
Bellehill Corp. national leader in geriatric rehab. seeks lic'd. P/T assistants to work in our East Bay facilities. F/T. $2000 signon bonus, $1000 continuing educ. bnft. $30K-$36K year. Exc bnfts. Send resume to: Joe Garcia, Farnam St., Oakland, CA 94601.

NURSING

LVN
Medical Assistant
Excellent opportunities in a dynamic multi-specialty medical clinic for individuals with 1 yr expr in an acute setting or back office environment. We offer excellent benefits & compensation.

Please send resume to: Personnel Dept., 253 N. Pastoria Ave., Louisville, KY 40223.

Sunny Brook
Medical Clinic

MEDICAL
**Lab Technologist**
Dade County is seeking a temporary per diem lab tech for the Public Health Division in Miami, Fl. Send resume: Dr. Marie Montgomery, 4823 Coco Palm Blvd., Miami, FL 33180. Equal Oppty. Employer.

### MEDICAL BOOKKEEPER

A/P, payroll, word processing, gen. ofc. Exp. pref. Flex. hrs. Sal. nego. Podiatry ofc.

Send resume: Personnel, 322 Fern Valley Way, Louisville, KY 40206.

### NURSING ASSISTANT

Beverly Manor is looking for a Certified/Non-Certified Nursing Assistant. AM/PM. Full-time shift. We offer certification classes. Please send resume:

**ADKINS MANOR**
1477 Grove Street
Philadelphia, PA 19124
Equal Opportunity Employer

**Medical Secretary/Asst.**
Heavy phones, good knowledge of medical terminology, light back office, organizational & peopleskills important. No bookkeeping, some typing. Send resume to: c/o Burton Job Network, P.O. Box 4718-767. York, PA 17403.

### DENTAL TEAM

Seeking an exceptional person for our progressive office. We value superior organizational & administrative skills and we focus on warmth caring & expert communication with our patients. Although previous experience in dentistry is not essential, we believe that applicants should be career minded, personally stable & health centered in their lifestyle. If you are searching for a real opportunity to grow and fulfill your potential, please see us. Send resume to Margaret A. Port, DDS - Orthodontist, 1855 San Miguel Dr., Redmond, WA 98055.

### CODING/ ABSTRACTING

Louisville's Madonna Hospital has a full-time opening for a Registered Records Administrator or an Accredited Record Technician. This person will be responsible for coding inpatient and outpatient records. Experience in ICD-9-CM coding required. We offer an excellent salary and benefit package. For more information, please send a resume to the Employment Manager.

MADONNA HOSPITAL
1401 W. Central Park
Louisville, KY 40223
Fax (502) 555-5863
Equal Opportunity Employer

## HOSPITAL OPPORTUNITIES

Liberty Hospital a progressive 132-bed facility, is offering the following opportunities:

★ Clerk Transcriber
Full time in Emergency Room, shift is negotiable.

★ Admitting Clerk
Full time, varied shifts.

For consideration, please send resume to our Personnel Dept., at LIBERTY HOSPITAL, 13855 E. 14th St., San Antonio, TX 78204.

### Liberty Hospital

**MEDICAL.** Chiropractic office seeks enthusiastic career oriented person to run Insurance Dept. Excellent opportunity for salary advancement. Small claims/insurance experience required. Send resume to: Howard Parker, P.O. Box 428, San Antonio, TX 78209, or Fax (210) 555-0877.

### DENTAL FRONT DESK

Do you have excellent communication skills over the phone & in person? Are you enthusiastic, caring & dependable? If you have exper. with appt. book control & bookkeeping & enjoy a challenge in a patient-centered practice, please send resume to: Gloria Sanchez, D.D.S., 4141 Port Royal Ct., Miami, FL 33157, or Fax (305) 555-8992.

**Occupational Therapist**
Montre-Ocean Senior Focus is seeking an enthusiastic Occupational Therapist with an interest in geriatrics and outpatient rehabilitation to join the health care team of the adult day health program and Comprehensive Outpatient Rehabilitation Facility.

This is a 20 hr./wk. position with flexible hours. Requires a BA in OT and AOTA certification.

We offer generous benefits. For immediate consideration, send your resume to: Employee Services, 1769 Lynhaven Rd., Ft. Worth, TX 76103. EOE.

Ⓜ **Montre-Ocean Hospitals**

Good Health from
Coast to Coast

ACTIVITY
WORKSHEETS

PORTFOLIO
UPDATE

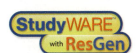

## Writing a Health Care Cover Letter

Review all of the newspaper health care employment ads in Figure 1.2.4. Select the job that is of most interest to you, and assume you have all of the qualifications. If you prefer, you may select an appropriate health care employment ad from your local newspaper. Then, remove the practice paper provided for Activity 5 in Section 3 and draft a cover letter. You may refer to the sample health care cover letters in this step when constructing your cover letter. Remember to look at the sample cover letter headings to decide where you want to include your address, telephone, and cell numbers with area code and your professional e-mail address. Use the same heading for your cover letter, resume, and reference list. After you have drafted your cover letter, show it to your instructor for evaluation. Make any necessary corrections. Then key your cover letter, saving it on the same thumb drive you used to store your resume. Print your final cover letter on 8 1/2 × 11 inch paper, the same grade and paper color used for your resume. Place your printed health care cover letter in your employment portfolio for future reference.

## StudyWARE™ Connection

Go to your software and complete the assessment activity to help you learn about a health care cover letter.

# Health Care Employment Application

## In this step you will find

- what health care employers want in an employment application.

- information needed to complete health care employment applications.

- a completed health care employment application to study.

- two blank health care employment applications to complete and use as references.

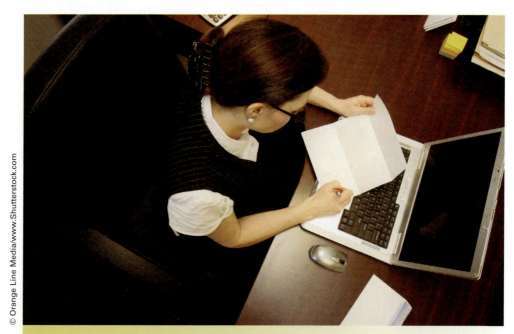

Your completed employment application will make it easier to fill out another one at an employer's job site or website.

## What Is a Health Care Employment Application?

Most health care employers require applicants to complete an employment application. See Figure 1.3.1 for an example of a completed health care employment application. Employment applications are health care facility documents that give the employer facts about you that can be kept on file. These facts include basic information on your education, skills, work history, and references. Even if you have a resume and a scheduled interview, you will usually need to complete an employment application form. You should be prepared to complete the form when you go online to a health care provider job site, on an interview, or when you make a cold call to a health care facility. Use the form you complete in this step as a guide for any of these occasions.

When you apply online to a health care provider you may be asked to create an account with a user name and password. You will complete and submit a profile or an application which you may use to apply for currently posted job openings.

**FIGURE 1.3.1** Application (Front)

# VALLEYCARE HEALTH CENTER

**EMPLOYMENT APPLICATION**

ValleyCare Health Center is an equal opportunity employer. This philosophy calls for equal opportunities for employment, training, and advancement regardless of sex, race, creed, color, age, national origin, religion, physical or mental handicap, or genetic information

*If possible, use a ball point pen for neatness and effect. (black ink preferred).*

*Follow directions.*

PRINT CLEARLY

## PERSONAL INFORMATION

DATE  JUNE 6, 20--    SOCIAL SECURITY NUMBER  825-56-0731

NAME  BROWN *(LAST)*    MICHAEL *(FIRST)*    J. *(MIDDLE)*

PRESENT ADDRESS  4852 STEVENSON RD *(STREET)*  HUNTINGTON *(CITY)*  OH *(STATE)*  45732 *(ZIP CODE)*

PERMANENT ADDRESS  SAME *(STREET)*  *(CITY)*  *(STATE)*  *(ZIP CODE)*

TELEPHONE NO.  (740) 555-0135    CELL NO. (740) 555-7216  E-MAIL  mjbrown@gmail.com

CAN YOU, AFTER EMPLOYMENT, SUBMIT VERIFICATION OF YOUR LEGAL RIGHT TO WORK IN THE UNITED STATES?  CIRCLE ONE:  (YES)  NO    (IF YES, VERIFICATION WILL BE REQUIRED)

*Employees with little or no work experience should indicate "open". Experienced employees should write "negotiable, or "Neg". Negotiable means that you would like to talk about the wage you have in mind.*

## EMPLOYMENT DESIRED

POSITION  MEDICAL RECORDS TECHNICIAN    DATE YOU CAN START  JUNE 15, 20--    SALARY DESIRED  OPEN

ARE YOU EMPLOYED NOW?  YES    IF SO MAY WE INQUIRE OF YOUR PRESENT EMPLOYER  YES

AVAILABILITY:  (DAYS)  (NIGHTS)  (PMS)  (WEEKENDS)  (FULL TIME)  (PART TIME)

| EDUCATION | NAME AND LOCATION OF SCHOOL | DEGREE OR CERTIFICATE OR LICENSE | SUBJECTS STUDIED |
|---|---|---|---|
| HIGH SCHOOL | WOODWARD H.S. | HIGH SCHOOL | GENERAL |
| | HUNTINGTON, OH | DIPLOMA | EDUCATION |
| UNIVERSITY OR COLLEGE | HUNTINGTON COLLEGE | A.A. DEGREE | ANATOMY, PHYSIOLOGY |
| | HUNTINGTON, OH | | MED. TERMINOLOGY |
| TRADE, BUSINESS, OR CORRESPONDENCE SCHOOL | | | |

*Write out full school names, no abbreviations.*

LIST SPECIAL SKILLS, QUALIFICATIONS, AND PERSONAL QUALITIES THAT APPLY TO THIS POSITION:
SPEAK SPANISH, DETAIL ORIENTED, SELF MANAGEMENT, GOOD TEAM SKILLS.

LIST WORKING KNOWLEDGE OF: COMPUTER SOFTWARE/EQUIPMENT/LANGUAGES:
KEY 80 W'PM, NDC MEDISOFT, IDX SYSTEMS, MICROSOFT WORD, E-CLINICAL WORKS.

LIST PROFESSIONAL ORGANIZATIONS:  N/A

*N/A shows you have read the statement or question and it does not apply to you.*

CONTINUED ON OTHER SIDE

LAST  FIRST  MIDDLE

**FIGURE 1.3.1** Application (Back)

WORK EXPERIENCE

Keep your reasons for leaving past jobs positive.

List all present and past employment, including part-time or seasonal, beginning with the most recent.

| Employer | Employment Dates and Salary | Describe the work you did in detail | Reason for leaving |
|---|---|---|---|
| Name  APPLIANCE PARTS<br><br>Address  435 BLACK AVE.<br><br>City  HUNTINGTON  State  OH, 45732<br><br>Phone (740) 555-0107  Supervisor  MR. OLIVER FORD | From:  MAY 15, 20--<br><br>To:  PRESENT<br><br>Starting Salary  12.00 HR<br><br>Ending Salary  13.50 HR | SALES<br>CASHIER<br>INVENTORY<br>DELIVERY<br>DISPLAY | START CAREER IN<br>HEALTH CARE |
| Name  YMCA SPORTS CAMP<br><br>Address  3071 ARTHUR AVE.<br><br>City  HUNTINGTON  State  OH, 45732<br><br>Phone (740) 555-0146 Supervisor  MR. JOHN NOWAK | From:  JULY 1, 20--<br><br>To:  AUG 15, 20--<br><br>Starting Salary  10.00 HR<br><br>Ending Salary  10.00 HR | COUNSELLOR<br>RESPONSIBLE<br>FOR CHILDREN<br>10-12<br>AEROBICS<br>PROGRAM DIRECTOR | SUMMER<br>EMPLOYMENT<br>ENDED |
| Name  MC DONALD'S RESTAURANT<br><br>Address  2437 SHOREVIEW<br><br>City  MINNEAPOLIS  State  MN, 55454<br><br>Phone (612) 555-0120 Supervisor MS. ANGELA CHACON | From:  NOV., 20--<br><br>To:  APRIL 30, 20--<br><br>Starting Salary  06.50 HR<br><br>Ending Salary  07.50 HR | COUNTER SALES<br>COOKING<br>CASHIER<br>MAINTENANCE | RELOCATION |

**REFERENCES:**
GIVE THE NAMES OF THREE PERSONS NOT RELATED TO YOU WHO CAN ATTEST TO YOUR EXPERIENCE AND QUALIFICATIONS.

| | NAME | BUSINESS NAME/ADDRESS | BUSINESS PHONE | OCCUPATION |
|---|---|---|---|---|
| 1 | MR. OLIVER FORD | APPLIANCE PARTS, 435 BLACK AVE. HUNTINGTON, OH, 45732 | (740) 555-0107 | MANAGER |
| 2 | MS. HEATHER MORENO | PATTERSON PRIZES, INC. 4721 HICKORY DRIVE HUNTINGTON, OH, 45732 | (740) 555-0134 | OWNER |
| 3 | MR. CHARLES BARABI | HUNTINGTON COLLEGE, 1045 PACIFIC AVE. HUNTINGTON, OH, 45732 | (740) 555-0182 | INSTRUCTOR |

I AUTHORIZE INVESTIGATION OF ALL STATEMENTS CONTAINED IN THIS APPLICATION. I UNDERSTAND THAT MISREPRESENTATION OR OMISSION OF FACTS CALLED FOR IS CAUSE FOR DISMISSAL. FURTHER, I UNDERSTAND AND AGREE THAT MY EMPLOYMENT IS FOR NO DEFINITE PERIOD AND MAY, REGARDLESS OF THE DATE OF PAYMENT OF MY WAGES AND SALARY, BE TERMINATED AT ANY TIME WITHOUT ANY PREVIOUS NOTICE.

When signing your application use your full name. Never use a nickname.

DATE  JUNE 6, 20--          SIGNATURE  *Michael Brown*

As a return user, you can view, update, or change your information. The employer may send you e-mail job alerts that match your qualifications. If your skills and experience appear to match an open position, a recruitment services professional or a hiring manager may contact you.

Be honest when you fill out a health care employment application. If you are hired and it is learned later that information on your application is untrue, you could be terminated for falsification of medical facility documents. For example, if you falsely claim to have a certification on your application and are subsequently hired, your manager might decide to fire you if he or she finds out about your deceit.

## What Do Health Care Employers Look for in an Employment Application?

The information you provide and how well you present the information creates an image of the type of employee you would be. The information indicates to a health care employer the following:

1. **Your ability to follow instructions.** Have you carelessly or carefully filled out the employment application? Keep it neat. Your application may also indicate how well you can read and write.

2. **Your ability to hold a health care job.** There will be questions concerning your employment history. You may be asked to explain gaps in employment.

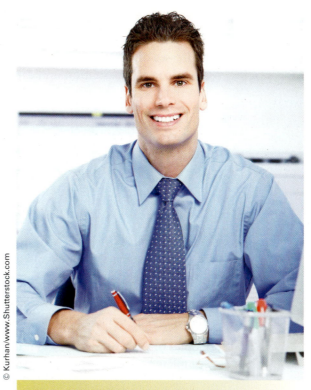

© Kurhan/www.Shutterstock.com

How well you complete a health care employment application could determine whether you are granted an interview.

3. **Your achievements.** The employment application allows you to mention past accomplishments. Mention specifically those related to health care.

4. **Your thoroughness.** Did you answer all the questions on the employment application? Don't leave blanks. Placing N/A (not applicable) shows the employer you have read the question and it does not apply to you.

Completing a health care employment application does not mean you will have an interview. The outcome could depend on how well you completed the employment application. *Remember*: Always include a copy of your resume with your employment application. A copy of your resume will help the hiring manager remember you.

## Completing a Health Care Employment Application

Carefully read the completed employment application for ValleyCare Health Center, Figure 1.3.1 in this step. Be sure to follow the side heading instructions, as they are very important for correctly completing an employment application. If a Social Security number is requested, you may choose to wait and give your Social Security number to an employer when you are hired. You may want to write on the application "Submit when hired." This is private information.

Make sure you have the following when completing a health care employment application:

1. Two pens (preferably black ink), two pencils, an eraser, paper clips.

2. Your current and previous addresses.

3. Education information, usually from high school to present. Give names and addresses of schools, the diplomas or degrees you earned, and the dates you attended each institution. Indicate any subjects, particularly those relating to health care and the job opening, in which you excelled.

4. Work records. Be able to provide the names, addresses, and phone numbers of past employers, the dates of employment, job responsibilities, the wages earned, the names of your supervisors, and your reasons for leaving each job. Keep your reasons for leaving a job positive. Include military experience (if any) and volunteer work.

5. List of your health care clinical, office, and equipment operation skills.

6. Names of certificates, licenses, professional organizations, and other medical-related documents, honors, and achievements that could give you an advantage over other applicants.

7. A list of references that shows names, job titles, health care facility names and company names, addresses, and telephone numbers.

8. Copies of your resume. Remember, if possible, attach your resume to any completed employment application.

# Activity 6

**ACTIVITY WORKSHEETS**

**WEBSITE**

**PORTFOLIO UPDATE**

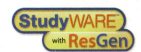

## Completing a Health Care Employment Application

Before you begin, review the completed sample application, Figure 1.3.1, in this step. Then gather the information and materials noted above. Be sure to have a copy of your resume because the application will require the same or similar information. First determine what health care job you are seeking. You need to be specific. The key is to think of a health care job title that you are most interested in or qualified for in the near future. If necessary, you can reference health care job titles on O*Net OnLine. You can also access the *Occupational Outlook Handbook,* the OOH, in your school career center, school or public library, or online at www.bls.gov/oco/. The ValleyCare Health Center is a very large medical organization. It has many job opportunities, including the health care position you want.

Remove Activity 6 in Section 3 and complete the first blank employment application for ValleyCare Health Center in pencil. When you have completed the employment application to your satisfaction, show it to your instructor for evaluation and then make any necessary corrections. Next, using your pencil draft, carefully complete the second ValleyCare Health Center employment application using a pen with black ink. This practice will help you complete employment applications in the future.

Then place your completed employment application in your employment portfolio. Use it as a reference when completing health care application forms in the future when you apply online or have an interview.

## StudyWARE™ Connection

Go to your software and play the Hangman game to help reinforce the health care employment application content discussed in this step.

### In this step you will find

- the definition of a job lead.

- how to prepare for job leads.

- ten sources of health care job leads.

- a method for researching a health care job and facility.

- an activity for recording health care job leads and contacts.

- an activity for researching a health care facility.

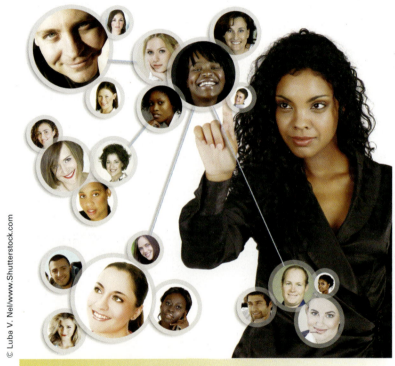

© Luba V. Nel/www.Shutterstock.com

Use the power of networking to find a health care job lead.

## What Is a Job Lead?

A job lead is a contact that may direct you to a job opening. The most promising job leads in health care may be found in the following ways:

- by contacting a school career center or placement office.

- by using your network of people to find health care job openings.

- by using the Yellow Pages to find health care employers to visit.

- by finding health care employment sources on the Internet.

- by acting on newspaper health care help-wanted ads.

Notice that each of the ways to find a job lead will take action on your part. The time and effort you spend looking for a job represents a considerable investment in your future. Finding the right job takes time, organization, and commitment.

## How Should You Prepare for Job Leads?

- **Be organized.** Make your job search effective. Establish a target date for getting a job. Decide how much time you will allow and be prepared for an extended search. If you are a student, start your job search months before you need a job. If you are unemployed, you should spend 8 hours every day (40 hours per week) on your job search—this *is* your job! Plan the minimum number of contacts you will make each day, or the minimum number of people to meet each day. Set daily and weekly goals for yourself. Use the system provided in Activity 7 for recording contacts and follow-up actions.

- **Have business cards made.** Giving a business card to prospective health care employers and networking contacts may be just the edge you need to be remembered when a job opening appears. A local print shop can prepare business cards for you—you need only to provide them with the proper information. Include your name, professional e-mail address, cell and/or telephone number, and job objective on the front of your business card. On the back, list your skills for your health care job objective. When you visit health care facilities that have no openings, ask if they would keep your business card on file. If they would like you to submit a resume, attaching your business card serves as a reminder of your visit. In fact, you may want to attach your business card along with your resume to **any** application form you complete. This will set your application apart from the others. See the example provided in Figure 1.4.1.

- **Plan your 15–30-second pitch.** Prepare what you will say to a person in your network who may find a job lead for you. You might say, "When I graduate I am looking for a job as _____. Do you know of someone I can contact about a job opening?" If you meet your contact personally, give him/her a business card.

### FIGURE 1.4.1 Business Card (Front and Back)

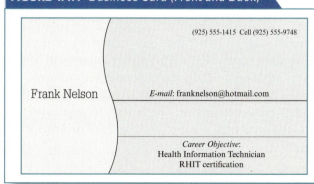

(925) 555-1415  Cell (925) 555-9748

Frank Nelson

*E-mail*: franknelson@hotmail.com

*Career Objective*:
Health Information Technician
RHIT certification

SKILLS:
Fox Meadows Accent Data Manager
eClinical Works software
Microsoft Access
Compliance with regulations
Detail orientated

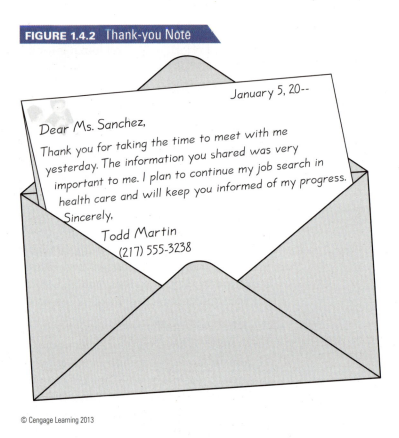

**FIGURE 1.4.2** Thank-you Note

January 5, 20--

Dear Ms. Sanchez,

Thank you for taking the time to meet with me yesterday. The information you shared was very important to me. I plan to continue my job search in health care and will keep you informed of my progress.

Sincerely,

Todd Martin
(217) 555-3238

© Cengage Learning 2013

- **Never overlook sending a thank-you note.** Buy note cards to write a thank-you to anyone who gave you a job lead, referred you to others who helped, or as a follow-up to a prospective employer. Send the thank-you note immediately after your contact. The note reaffirms your interest in the job and shows you are serious about your job search. The note should be legible, short, and grateful. You may want to e-mail your thanks, but a handwritten note often makes a greater impact. See the sample provided in Figure 1.4.2.

- **Find a mentor.** A mentor is someone who will give you encouragement, guidance, and support throughout your job search. Your mentor can be a parent, a relative, or someone whom you know well and trust. Try to find a mentor who has contacts in the town where you want to work. Check with your mentor often and seek advice.

# Proven Ways to Find Job Leads

There are many ways to get a health care job other than just scattering your resumes. You must do more than sending resumes and waiting for an answer. Make better use of your time. When you pursue job leads, many people get to know you and your medical career goals. Be aware, however, that trying several job lead techniques may not be as helpful as concentrating on only a few. To make sure your job search efforts are successful, you may want to choose three or four of the following job lead techniques:

**Job Lead 1: School Career Center or Placement Office.** School career centers and placement offices are excellent sources to contact for health care job opportunities. Placement counselors may offer other services, such as assisting you in resume and cover letter writing. You will be provided with an employment application to complete and file with your school career center and/or placement office. Your placement counselor will contact employers and provide a list of health care job openings. Ask the employment counselor to set up an interview for you.

**Job Lead 2: Networking.** It is estimated that up to 90% of jobs are found through networking. In fact, the more contacts you make, the better your chances of finding employment.

- Show people in your network a list of health care employers who you think would hire persons with your qualifications. Ask if they know anyone who works there, especially managers, that you could contact. Most people like helping others.

- People you see socially or in business in places you go every day may have a lead—you just have to let them know about the health care job you want! Ask them if they have any advice or suggestions about your job search. Ask them if they know of any potential contacts in politics, banking, real estate, or service clubs such as Rotary, Lions Club, or Kiwanis. Someone may be able to assist you in speaking to those persons about your job search.

- Going to job fairs, volunteering, or taking a health care class will also expand your network. Contact is best face-to-face, but do not forget to call or e-mail people whom you have not seen for a while.

- Engage in social media, but make sure you keep your Twitter account and your profiles and pages on Facebook and LinkedIn professional. Be prepared that a potential employer may look you up on these accounts and may Google you. A potential employer may view your postings as representing how you will communicate with health care employees. Your postings should reflect a mature, ethical attitude. If you have any questionable posts on these public sites, it could cost you a job you do not even have yet. To minimize this, you should use social media privacy settings. Add recommendations from supervisors to your profiles. Join a medical group in your health care specialty to connect with other health care professionals. Your social network can help you identify health care hiring managers, research health care facilities and their job openings, and stay current on health care industry news.

- Networking may help you find jobs that are not advertised. Health care employers often hire from recommendations their employees tell them about. It may be that the person who gives you a lead may not know you at all. It could be a friend of a friend of a friend. This is the power of networking. The more contacts you make, the better your chances of finding employment. Your contact list may include the following:

| family | teachers | doctors |
|---|---|---|
| friends | counselors | team members |
| parents | church members | dentist |
| students | club members | salespersons |
| real estate people | bankers | barber/hairdresser |
| relatives | advisors | waiters/waitresses |
| neighbors | coaches | |
| business people | co-workers | |

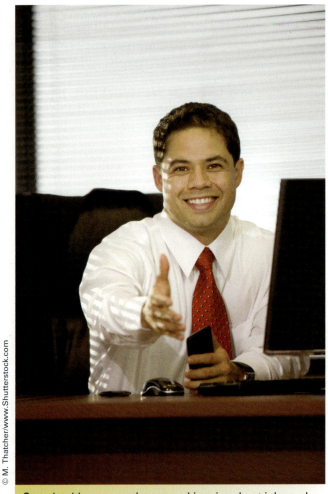

© M. Thatcher/www.Shutterstock.com

Go to health care employers and inquire about jobs and their application process.

Give people who offer to help you a copy of your business card and, if appropriate, a copy of your resume. Keep in touch by calling or e-mail, and keep a record of your contacts on the forms provided in Activity 7. By following up with your contacts, your request is a reminder that you are still looking for work. Your contacts are more likely to inquire about job leads for you when they talk to their friends or people they know in business. They may hear about a job opening before it becomes public and may agree to act as a reference for you.

- Health care job fairs are mainly held for health care organizations to attract new hires. Attending job fairs is a casual way of coming face-to-face with employer contacts. Remember to dress as if you are going to a job interview, and bring copies of your resume and business card. Human resource personnel often attend job fairs, hoping to hire enthusiastic new employees. At job fairs, you can get inside information such as what health care employers are looking for and who to contact (by picking up business cards). You can also obtain employment applications. Job fairs are advertised in the newspaper or on health care employer websites.

**Job Lead 3: Market Survey.** One of the most successful ways to find a job is by calling or visiting health care employers and asking if they have any job openings. Use the local business *Yellow Pages* index to make a list of all the health care organizations that you want to contact to see if they have an opening for the job in which you are trained. You may be attracted to a health care facility because you have heard it is a good place to work. To find what you should know about the health care organization before your contact, read the section "Researching a Health Care Facility" in this step. If you want a job in a different town, use the Internet *Yellow Pages* site, www.yellowpages.com.

Here are tips for contacting employers whether they have an opening or not.

- Rather than calling, walk right in. Ask for the human relations or human resource office or for a small health care facility, whoever is in charge of hiring. Ask if the health care facility is hiring for your type of position. You may be able to make an appointment, or be interviewed immediately. Once you have met the hiring person face-to-face, you might be remembered when there is an opening! Armed with your resume and business card, give your pitch.

Introduce yourself and say, "Hello, I am _____ and a student at _____. I am interested in working in a health care facility such as this one. I will graduate soon as a _____. Is there someone I can talk to about a job opening?"

Always ask if you may leave your resume and business card, and be sure to check back often. Send a thank-you note.

- If you are considering a few health care facilities, prepare and send a different cover letter to each. Be sure to find something specific to say about each organization. (Read the section "Researching a Health Care Facility" in this step for assistance.) For example, you might explain what it is about the health care organization that appeals to you or what it does that you feel is important. If you do not hear back within a short time, call, e-mail, or stop in to get an interview.

After you contact a health care employer, remember to send a thank-you note and stay in touch by contacting periodically to see if there are any openings. It is good to contact more than once a health care facility for which you would like to work. This shows your enthusiasm and interest in the organization.

**Job Lead 4: Internet Job Listings.** Many of the sources of job leads presented in this step can be accessed through the Internet. Here are some other good ways you can search online job listings:

- Search for a job through the websites of specific health care facilities in which you are interested. Use your favorite search engines such as Google or Yahoo and key the employer's name in the search box. On the company home page, you should find links such as "Career Opportunities," or "Job Openings" which will connect you to information about careers with the organization. Health care employer websites post available full-time and part-time jobs, company profiles, lists of upcoming job fairs, and directions for completing a profile and/or posting your resume. One of the advantages of creating your information profile online with a health care organization is that your information gets into the system immediately. When the health care organization reviews your information they look for the best match for the position based on the qualifications they listed in the job posting. If your skills and experience appear to match an open position, a recruitment services professional or a hiring manager may contact you. Be sure to keep your profile current and check your e-mail and phone messages as they may contact job candidates by either method.

- Search health care job boards or general ones that compile health care job postings from other sources such as other job boards, newspapers' job sections, company career pages, recruiter sites, and more. Usually you will find contacts for applying to available jobs by state and area with directions for applying online. Some of the proven Internet sites are:

| | |
|---|---|
| www.Careerbuilder.com | www.Job-hunt.org |
| www.HealthEcareers.com | www.MedZilla.com |
| www.Healthjobsusa.com | www.Monster.com |
| www.hotjobs.yahoo.com | www.Simplyhired.com |
| www.Indeed.com | |

**Job Lead 5: Newspaper Employment Ads.** Do not forget one of the common sources of job leads. The health care want ads and the business section in your local newspaper can help you find a job.

WEBSITE

- Read the health care help-wanted ads in your local newspaper regularly. The Sunday newspaper is where most job postings appear, but also check the daily edition for a job that may be posted there first. Promptly send a specific resume and cover letter to each health care address for which you may be qualified. Carefully tailor your resume and cover letter to the job requirements in the ad.

- Almost all newspapers of any size now have their own Internet job boards and post their help-wanted ads. The online ads usually have posting dates and an easy application process. The American Journalism Review's NewsLink, www. newslink.org, is an online listing of newspapers sorted by state. You can access the help-wanted ads in the newspaper you select and contact them or apply online.

- Newspapers may have ads for a Virtual Job Fair, their local newsgroup online job search site. You can access their website for local health care facility job postings and complete an information profile and upload your resume.

- Read the business section of your local newspaper for health care organizations reporting business plans, expansions, and new locations. Watch for news stories about physicians' offices and small health care facilities creating more jobs. You will learn about the community and health care employers to contact.

**Job Lead 6: Associations.** Membership in a medical association offers a career advantage. Many associations have inexpensive student memberships. Some publish informative magazines that include employment want ads. These associations can help you become familiar with certifications and may offer job alert e-mail. They offer face-to-face networking opportunities through meetings, job fairs, and conferences where "job talk" is always prevalent.

- Check your local library for the *Encyclopedia of Associations,* which lists professional medical associations. Look up the association for your health care job to find their website, telephone and fax numbers, and e-mail and postal address.

- If your library subscribes to the Gale database, access it through your library website and click "Associations Unlimited" and your professional medical association. You will link to the association home page and find contact, conference, and employment information.

- Using your favorite search engine, key "Association of" or "American Medical" and your job title, for your association website.

**Job Lead 7: U.S. Federal Government.** For health care jobs with the U.S. federal government, use their official job site, USAJOBS, at www.usajobs.gov. This website updates health care job openings, including locations, duties, salaries, and complete employment instructions, including how to submit an application. The vacancy announcements will indicate if a specific written test is necessary. Jobs with the federal government are competitive with the private sector; if you add their benefits to the salaries, government jobs often come out ahead.

- The U.S. Department of Veterans Affairs is a leader in U.S. health care and has a wide range of health care employment opportunities with incentive programs in their hospitals and clinics. Go to www.va.gov/jobs/ to contact human relations office personnel by state and area to obtain information about health care job vacancies, and download an application.

**Job Lead 8: One-Stop Career Centers.** These career centers are located throughout the nation and are government sponsored through the U.S. Department of Labor. To locate the nearest One-Stop Career Center, check the telephone business listings, or go online at www.servicelocator.org. They offer free job and career resources, including computers, fax, career advising, resume help, and local job listings. Access their website, www.careeronestop.org and select the job search links for career information and to locate health care employer websites by state and region.

**Job Lead 9: Private Employment Agencies.** Private employment agencies are listed under "Employment Agencies" in the *Yellow Pages*. Contact private employment agencies and find the ones who provide health care employment. Ask them for a screening and an interview. Give them a copy of your resume. They also provide job leads, career counseling, and assistance with resume writing and interview techniques. Deal only with an employment agency that has a good reputation. Some employment agencies charge you a fee for their services; others charge the employer with whom they found you a job. The latter tend to be for high-level jobs. Normally the employment agency will want you to sign an employment contract. Be sure you understand the requirements and cost, if any, of the contract before signing. Research thoroughly, and do not use an agency if you cannot find anyone to recommend it. Be sure the agency really has something to offer that you could not find elsewhere.

**Job Lead 10: Temporary Employment Agencies.** Temporary employment agencies are listed under "Employment" or "Employment—Temporary" in the *Yellow Pages*. Their listings or ads will usually tell what their specialties are. You may want a temporary health care job simply to get work experience. Temporary jobs can last from a few hours to several months. Many health care employers need extra help for special projects and to fill in for employees who are on vacation or taking a leave of absence. Temporary employment may lead to a permanent job. These temporary health care experiences can help you make sound medical employment decisions.

## Researching a Health Care Job

WEBSITE

If you are planning on a particular health care job, you can learn more about it by using the O*Net OnLine website. O*Net OnLine is continually updated and provides the latest career trends and job information. The information comes from the computerized database of O*Net developed under the U.S. Department of Labor. Learning to use O*Net OnLine will help you in your work life. The research for your health care job will help you write your resume and cover letter and complete an employment application, as well as perfect your interviewing skills. In the future, you may want to explore related jobs in the health care field.

You should know the answers to the following questions about a health care job before you go for an interview:

- What are the skills and knowledge needed in this job?

- What are the tasks, tools, and technologies required in this job?

- What are the work styles and work values important to this job?

Now, go online to the O*Net OnLine.org home page and click "Find Occupations." Key in your job title and you will be linked to detailed information about it. Next, print the pages that describe your job. Then, find the following categories for your health care job: Tasks, Tools, Knowledge, Skills, Abilities, and Work Activities. Read the information in each of these categories, and using a marker or pen, highlight the requirements in each category that you want to focus on and/or develop at this time. Next, find the categories Work Styles and Work Values. Read the personal characteristics listed in these categories and highlight one quality in each category that you find important to you in a health care job.

PORTFOLIO
UPDATE

This job information will give you a clear picture of what is expected in your health care job. Finally, place the O*Net printout of your health care job information in your employment portfolio to use as a reference for your future health care employment.

## Researching a Health Care Facility

Do not make the mistake of following up a job lead without knowing something about the health care facility. Research will give you an idea if this is the health care facility that really appeals to you. When you call or walk in and make your pitch, you will be able to say what impresses you about the organization if you have researched it beforehand. Health care employers like to hear something good about their organization, and what you say will show your interest in them. You do not want to appear that you are just contacting this lead at random. If you know something about the organization and their services, you will improve your chances of being considered

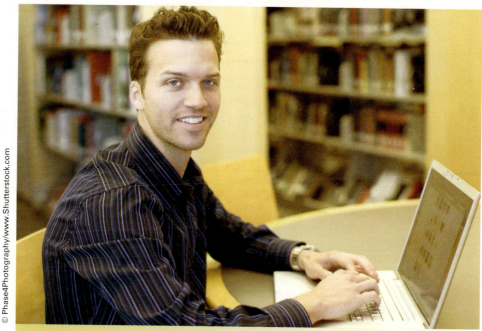
Research a health care employer before you interview.

for an interview. To find out more about a specific health care facility you can do the following:

- Talk to people who work there. Ask them what services the health care facility provides, and what it is like to work there.

- Write or call the health care facility for information. Explain that you are interested in learning about the services they provide. Tell them that you want to learn what their mission statement is, how it got started, and what important things have recently happened in the health care facility to improve its services.

WEBSITE

- Use the Internet. Check the health care facility website for information on its mission, philosophy, and services. Read and download the health care facility annual report. Look for the latest information about what is new. See how the health care facility describes itself so that you can focus your cover letter on the organization's interests. Print the pages that interest you.

- Go to the library. Ask the reference librarian to help you find the best resources for your research.

You should know as much about a health care facility as you can before you visit, send out a resume, or go for an interview. Answers to these questions will provide the most important information:

1. What services does this health care facility provide?

2. What kinds of health care jobs do they have?

3. In what cities does this health care organization have facilities?

4. How large is this health care facility?

5. Is the health care facility growing or shrinking in number of employees?

6. What are the health care facility's plans for the future?

7. Who are this health care facility's competitors?

After you have researched and done your best to answer the preceding questions about the organization, there may still be some questions you were not able to answer. These are the questions you may want to ask at a health care job interview. Also, consider any other questions that you have thought of as a result of your research. Asking good questions will show your interest and enthusiasm for the job.

## Activity 7

**ACTIVITY WORKSHEETS**

**PORTFOLIO UPDATE**

### Finding Health Care Job Leads

Carefully examine each source of health care job leads presented in this step. Decide on the sources you want to use and three or four leads you wish to pursue. For each health care facility, record the source you used and the name of the person who gave you the lead (if applicable). Then record the name of the health care facility, your contact and their title, the date, telephone number, e-mail address if available, mailing address, and any notes you may have on your conversation with them. Remove the forms provided in Section 3 for Activity 7. Keeping track of your health care contacts during your job search gives an accurate record of where you applied for a job and where you want to follow up. When you have completed your job leads to your satisfaction, show them to your instructor for evaluation. Place all vital job lead information in your employment portfolio.

## Activity 8

**ACTIVITY WORKSHEETS**

**PORTFOLIO UPDATE**

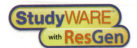

### Researching a Health Care Facility

A visit to your school library or career center, local library, health care facility, or health care facility website will likely be necessary to complete this activity. Remove Activity 8 in Section 3. Select and research one to three health care facilities for this activity. Record your answers to the research questions for each of your health care facilities. When you have completed your research paper to your satisfaction, show it to your instructor for evaluation. Then place it in your employment portfolio as a guide for researching a health care facility in the future.

### StudyWARE™ Connection

Go to your software and watch Carl's video and Robin's introduction and interview and answer the questions relating to the importance of research before a health care interview.

### In this step you will find

- a discussion of four important ways to prepare for a health care interview.

- a checklist to help you prepare for a health care interview.

- 12 of the most common interview questions and their appropriate responses.

- a list of questions you should consider concerning the job opening and the health care facility.

- an activity to help you answer 12 of the most common interview questions.

## Why Is Personal Preparation Important?

Congratulations, you have an interview. Your hard work has paid off. Your cover letter and resume have convinced a prospective employer to interview you for a health care position. Now you need to prepare yourself for a successful job interview. Personal preparation for an interview is important. Being well prepared before the interview increases your self-confidence. Making a good first impression on the interviewer helps the interviewer determine if you make a good fit with their health care team. If you are well groomed, and your attire is business-like, your image will show respect and show that you care about the job. You will inspire the interviewer to have confidence in your qualifications.

Your goals at that interview will be to learn more about the job, convince the employer you are the right person for the job, and gather enough information about the health care facility and job to determine if you want the position, if it is offered.

## What to Do before a Health Care Interview

1. **Find out as much as you can about the health care facility.** Some people have accepted job offers only to find that the work, the health care facility, and the services were not what they expected. These people did not adequately research the employer, nor did they ask the right questions at the interview. If you did not research the health care facility before responding to a job lead, you should do so before you have your interview. Reread the section on researching a company in Section 1, Step 4, and follow the guidelines there. At a minimum, you should know what services the health care facility offers and what kinds of jobs it provides. Prepare a question from the information you find from your research, and be ready to ask it during the interview. For example:

   "According to your website information, this health care facility is now rated as one of the top five in the state. How have patient outcomes been improved?"

   "*The Times Globe* states that plans are underway to double the size of this health care facility. What services will be added or expanded with this program?"

You will make a great impression in the interview if you relate what you know about the health care facility. You should tell what impresses you about the facility and what you find most interesting.

2. **Review the health care job description.** In an interview, you will want to describe how your qualifications relate to those required in the health care job. Use the copy you made of your job information from O*Net, or obtain a copy of the job description from the health care facility website. Prepare to describe to the interviewer how your skills and experience relate to the health care job and how you will be able to perform the tasks the job requires. Give a real life experience telling how you have used these skills in a job, clinical internship, or learned them in a class at school.

3. **Be organized.** You now have your employment portfolio. You should bring all the material you need for the health care interview in it to the interview. This includes another copy of your resume, your cover letter, your reference list, a completed employment application, and a copy of the job description. Organize this material and any other information you need in your employment portfolio. You will also want to arrive 10 to 15 minutes early. Take a practice drive and allow for delays. Organize clothes that you will wear to your job interview that give you a professional image. You will want to dress conservatively. Wear subdued solid colors. Men cannot go wrong with a crisp, collared, white, long-sleeved shirt, tailored suit pants, coordinating dark socks, and shined leather shoes. Add a tie and business jacket if it is the standard for the health care facility. For women, a jacket, tailored blouse, slacks or knee-length skirt, with plain leather pumps, is the dress code in many health care settings. Before the interview, review and use Figure 1.5.1, the Interview Checklist. Use these tips to help you make a good impression at the interview.

4. **Think about questions you will be asked and how to answer them.** You may be asked to provide more detail on information provided in your resume or application. There are many possible questions that may be asked during a health care interview. Of these, the 12 questions that follow—or some variation of them—are among the most common. Prepare yourself for your own interview by reading these questions and speaking their suggested answers. Keep in mind the suggested answers are examples of good businesslike responses. Consider what makes each response a good one. Whenever you have an interview, read and rehearse these questions with a specific health care facility and job in mind. Then prepare and *practice, practice, practice* verbalizing your answers until you feel comfortable and sound confident.

# Twelve of the Most Common Interview Questions

1. **Why are you interested in this health care position?** When you respond to this question, be specific. State the education and applicable skills you have.

"Because I am good at keying, scheduling appointments, and all jobs related to medical office work, I would be an excellent front office medical assistant."

"I am experienced in the care and use of EKG equipment and in preparing patients for the EKG series. I am familiar with EKG safety precautions, and all other work related to being an EKG technician."

**FIGURE 1.5.1** Interview Checklist

## Interview Checklist

Post and read this checklist one week before the interview to remind yourself what you need to do. Reread it the night before the interview. Place a check mark (✓) beside each item as you complete it.

### When Interview Is Scheduled

☐ Review your research or research the health care facility.

☐ Prepare a card with the time and place of the interview and the name of the interviewer. Mark the date and time in your calendar.

☐ Get directions to the interview location. A practice run may be helpful.

### Day Before the Interview

- **Gather the following supplies in your Employment Portfolio or briefcase:**

☐ Two pens and two pencils for filling out forms at the interview

☐ Money for parking, lunch, etc.

☐ Resume

☐ Completed employment application from Step 3. Use it as a reference when completing the company's employment application.

☐ Samples of your work (keyboarding samples, diagrams, etc.)

☐ Military records

☐ Social Security number

☐ Diplomas and special training certificates

☐ Licenses—driver's license or other special licenses

☐ Reference letters or list

☐ Other papers or materials that will help you obtain employment

- **Plan your appearance:**

☐ Check to see if you need a haircut.

☐ Lay out clothes you are to wear. Check that they are clean, mended, pressed, and a conservative style in subdued solid colors.

☐ Polish shoes. Make sure heels are not worn.

### Day of the Interview

- **Check your appearance:**

☐ Hair is washed and neatly styled.

☐ Body is bathed; deodorant is used.

☐ Minimal make-up and jewelry, and no perfume or after-shave lotion.

☐ Fingernails are neatly trimmed and clean.

☐ Teeth are clean; breath is fresh.

### Going to the Interview

☐ Leave for the interview early. Take the card with the directions and phone number with you.

☐ Go alone to the interview.

☐ Be polite in the outer office.

☐ Know the name(s) and title(s) of the person(s) who will interview you.

☐ Allow enough time for the interview.

"I am dedicated to providing the best possible patient experience. The challenge of this licensed vocational nursing position is exciting."

2. **We need a reliable person for this health care position. Can we rely on you?**
This question may concern handling the health care job stress, following the policies and procedures, and also regular work attendance. You might clarify the question, then say:

"It is very important to me to keep myself physically fit for the demands of a health care job."

"The physical well-being of patients is foremost in my plan to know the hospital policies and follow procedures exactly. Also, I aim to do my part to help this hospital maintain high safety standards."

"I am responsible and will be here as scheduled. While training and attending classes to be a medical assistant, I didn't miss a session."

3. **What pay do you expect?** Know what the pay range is for the health care position you want before the interview. You may find this out from the health care facilities employment office or from the original job ad. The health care ad may include some clues to the salary range. "No Experience Necessary" suggests a salary at the low end of the range. If no salary information is available, find out what the salary range is for that type of health care work. If you do not know what the range is, ask. You may also say you are open to suggestion or ask if the salary is negotiable.

"Considering my experience, what is the hourly pay range for this health care job?"

"I understand that the annual salary range for this position is $27,000–$35,000. Based on the responsibilities you've described and my experience, I believe $30,000 would be appropriate."

4. **Why do you want to work for our health care facility?** To answer this question, obtain as much information as you can about the health care facility before attending the interview. If possible, obtain a mission statement and information about the types of health services, working conditions, work environment, career opportunities, and responsiveness to patients' needs. This information might come from your health care facility research as described in Step 4, from people who work for the health care employer, from past employees, from patients who use its services, from persons who are familiar with the health care industry, and even from your own observation and judgment. Your efforts will show that you are seriously interested in working for the health care facility. This information will allow you to discuss the health care facility intelligently. Note the following responses:

"Your health care organization has one of the largest research programs in the United States and contributes to medical knowledge worldwide. I want to be part of a health care organization that is on the leading edge of innovation."

"I learned the founding principle of this health care organization is not just to address sickness, but your mission is to practice preventive medicine. I respect that you provide health education programs to optimize the health of patients."

5. **Have you had any serious illness or injury that might prevent you from performing your duties in this health care position?** The response to this question is easy if there has been no problem. However, if in the past you had a medical problem or injury, be prepared to show a clearance slip from your physician. The clearance slip should state that you are physically able to perform the health care job you are seeking. If you have no physical problem, you might say:

"No, I am in excellent health and can perform all duties required as a dental assistant."

However, if you had a problem in the past, the following answer would be appropriate:

"At this time, I can perform all of the duties of a surgical technologist. My medical problem in the past has been corrected and here is my physician's clearance slip."

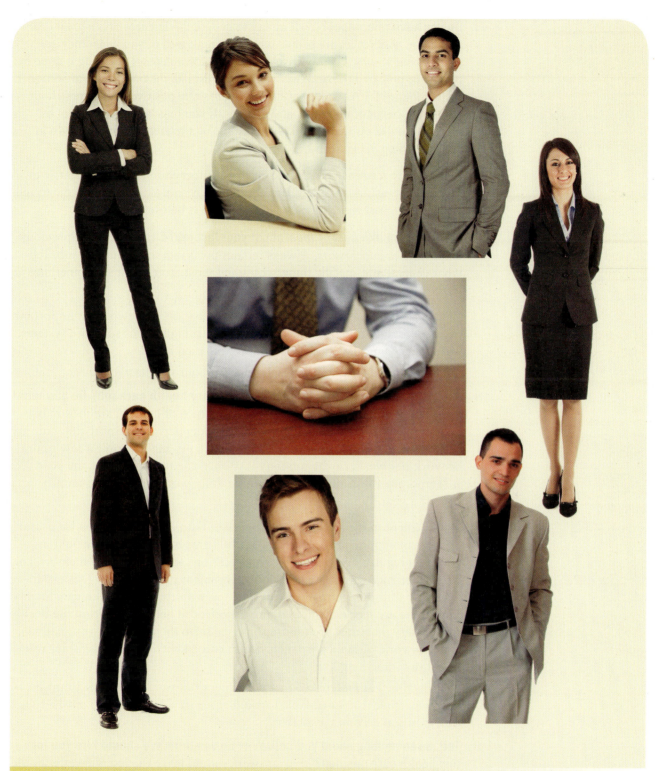

Look like a professional while searching for a health care job. Plan what you will wear and your appearance before the health care interview. Grooming is an important component.

Source: Clockwise from top left: © Maridav/www.Shutterstock.com; © Yuri Arcurs/www.Shutterstock.com; © Kharidehal Abhirama Ashwin/www. Shutterstock.com; © Minerva Studio/www.Shutterstock.com; © Netfalls/www.Shutterstock.com; © Skripko Ievgen/www.Shutterstock.com; © Andresr/www.Shutterstock.com; Middle image: © Offscreen/www.Shutterstock.com

6. **Do you have references?** Your ability to get good references says a great deal about you. References are people who will speak well of you when they are asked about you by a prospective employer. Most reference checking is done by phone. Be prepared to hand over a reference list like the one shown in Section 1, Step 1, Figure 1.1.6. A reference letter is generally positive statements about your character, attitude, skills, and abilities. If you have a reference letter, be prepared to discuss that as well. An example of a reference letter is shown in Section 2, Step 3, Figure 2.3.1.

"Here is my reference list. Mrs. Smith, my supervisor, is very familiar with my medical insurance billing and coding internship skills. She told me to tell you that the best time to reach her by phone is before noon."

7. **What did you like *best* or *least* about your last job?** Do not criticize previous employers or supervisors. Always remain positive about your last job. Tell what general and specific things you liked most. You might say something like:

"There were many things I liked about my last job. The two most important items were the people I worked with and learning various software systems, including eClinicalWorks, which I'm told is used here."

Do not respond to things you did not like about your last job.

8. **Are you looking for a permanent or temporary health care job? Do you want full-time or part-time work?** The time structure of health care jobs may be temporary part-time, temporary full-time, permanent part-time, or permanent full-time. A temporary part-time job may involve a few hours of work per week, or the job may last only one month during the year. A temporary full-time job may involve daily work for a week, month, or half a year.

A permanent part-time job would be fewer than 35 hours a week for a year or more of employment. A permanent full-time health care job would involve the regular 40-hour week with vacations and holidays. Remember, you gain experience with a temporary or permanent part-time job. This experience may lead to a permanent full-time job with the same health care facility. Employers are more inclined to hire experienced help from within the health care facility than they are to hire someone from the outside. If you really want to work within a particular health care facility try to be flexible. You might say something like:

"At this time I am interested in a permanent full-time nursing assistant position, but if one is not available I would agree to a part-time job until a full-time position becomes available."

9. **Tell me something about yourself. Why do you think we should hire you for this health care position?** Your answers should leave the interviewer with the right picture of you. You should describe your personal characteristics that will contribute to the job. You might say:

"I give my wholehearted effort to whatever I do. I look forward to using my medical office skills working with your storage and retrieval systems."

Keep your answer to why you should be hired on a professional level. Discuss only those traits that relate to the health care job. Be specific.

Give an example that will show how your educational background, internships, work experience, and any skills, interests, and hobbies you have would make you the best choice for the job.

"I can bring to the job excellent accounting skills from the billing software, QMSoftware Receivables Management system I learned at Los Positas College."

"In school I was on the softball team. I enjoyed that experience and learned the importance of working with diversity as a team member."

"I can think critically when listening to patients. I can eliminate unnecessary information and pay attention to the heart of the problem."

10. **How well do you work under pressure?** Almost all jobs in health care have some stress and require a worker to meet deadlines. To give a positive answer to this question you might say:

"From my clinical internship experience I know health care work can be stressful. I feel it is necessary to focus on remaining calm in a high-stress situation and keep my emotions in check."

"My present schoolwork requires me to meet deadlines. I manage and organize my work to meet these deadlines without undue pressure. I have never missed a deadline."

11. **What are your strengths and weaknesses?** Describe your strengths. This shows confidence and a positive attitude. If possible, do not discuss any weakness you might have. Sell yourself; modesty will not win you a job. Be prepared to back up statements with past examples. Possible strengths might be:

"I learn new skills quickly. On my last job I became proficient in Microsoft Windows 7 and front office procedures within a week."

"I work well under pressure. With Baxter Medical I never missed a monthly billing deadline."

"I am thorough with my class assignments. I pride myself on being aware of details in my day-to-day tasks."

If the interviewer presses you to describe a weakness, use the following suggestions to turn a weakness into a strength:

"I'm a perfectionist. I do not feel comfortable handing over a job that is less than the best I can do—even if it means working on it on my own time."

"Some co-workers think I am too organized. But I find it really saves time in the long run if I budget time each day for part of a big project so I can meet the deadline."

12. **What are your short-term and long-term health care employment goals?** A safe short-term goal answer might be:

"My goal is to become a productive health care employee in a short period of time. I am eager to learn all I can about respiratory therapy as a C.R.T. and the health care field."

A safe long-term goal answer might be:

"My long-term goal is to become a true health care professional and team member as a registered respiratory therapist. I would like to obtain my Registered Respiratory Therapist (R.R.T.) credential."

There are, of course, hundreds of potential questions. Some other common interview questions include:

How would you describe yourself working as a member of a team?

Tell me about your education.

Tell me about an achievement of which you are most proud.

Tell me about a time when you encountered a difficult situation. What happened and how did you handle it?

Take each question as an opportunity to talk about your skills and strengths and to learn more about the requirements of the job for which you are applying.

# Getting Answers to Your Employment Questions

Your work represents one of the most time-consuming aspects of your life. Decisions about a health care job offer should always be made with care and research. There are many important questions you will want answered *before* accepting a health care job offer. These questions and their answers come from the following:

- Your research of the job opening and health care facility.
- Your observation of the health care workplace.
- Information provided during the interview.
- Questions you ask during the interview.

By researching the job and the health care facility thoroughly before the interview, you will be prepared to ask questions that could determine whether you would in fact enjoy the job the facility has to offer. Asking good questions indicates to the employer that you are an intelligent, informed candidate for the position.

Carefully read the following questions about *you* and the job opening and *you* and the health care facility. Go to your interview armed with the answers to some of these questions from the research you did. Once at the health care facility you will be able to see the workplace from the inside. You will have a better sense from the work environment of whether or not you will be happy working there. During the interview, listen carefully for some of the following questions to be answered. At the end of the interview you will likely have an opportunity to ask questions. Be prepared to ask one or two questions that you have prepared from your research, or from observation of the workplace, or from information you heard in the interview, or from questions that were not answered and are appropriate to ask.

Remember, the answers to these questions may give you the information you need to make a very important life decision—accepting a job you will love.

## You and the Health Care Job Opening

- Why is there a health care job opening?
- Where have others who have held this job been reassigned within the health care facility?

- In addition to the duties and responsibilities listed in the health care job description, are there any other requirements or commitments I should know about?

- How and when is a new health care employee to be evaluated?

- Does the health care employee evaluation system seem fair?

- Is the health care position challenging or will it be boring work as time goes on?

- What training can a new health care employee expect?

- Will there be an employee probationary period (a trial period before becoming a permanent health care employee)?

- Is the physical health care work environment clean, well decorated, and properly maintained?

Add any other questions that you would like to have answered.

_____

_____

_____

## You and the Health Care Facility

- How does the health care facility's employee wage and benefit package compare with others in the same industry?

- What is the employee turnover rate at this health care facility?

- What are some of the health care facility's new services?

- What is the health care employer's reputation in the community and in the industry?

- How are health services offered by the organization rated in the field?

- How will the health care employer's policies and procedures affect you?

- How will the health care employer's work expectations and work hours affect your private life?

Add any other questions that you would like to have answered.

_____

_____

## Interview Killer Questions

Generally speaking, you should not start a discussion about salary or wages. Let the interviewer initiate this conversation. Job seekers should not ask certain questions during an interview because they may seem inappropriate or insensitive. For example: How much will I make? What days do I get off? How much vacation time do I get? How many paid holidays do I get? How much sick leave do I get?

These questions are self-serving. More concern is shown for *getting out of work* than for *getting a job*. Although the questions are important, they usually will be answered before you need to ask. This kind of information is a normal part of any serious interview.

## Activity 9.1

### Answering Interview Questions

To begin this exercise, identify a specific job at a specific health care facility for which you would like to interview. You may want to use the job you researched on O*Net or the health care facility you researched in Step 4. Then remove the worksheets for Activities 9.1 and 9.2 in Section 3. Write your answers to the 12 common interview questions. You may refer to the answers provided in this manual when writing your answers. Writing responses to interview questions helps you keep the answers in your mind so you will not be caught off guard in an interview. When you have answered the questions to your satisfaction, show them to your instructor for evaluation.

## Activity 9.2

### Practice Interview Evaluation Form

Work in groups of three. Have one person act as the interviewer and ask each question. Answer them with your written replies. Have a third person listen and complete Activity 9.2, the "Practice Interview Evaluation Form." After the interview, discuss your performance using the evaluation results, then switch roles. If you practice answering the questions before you attend the actual interview, your confidence will definitely increase. Put your answers to the interview questions and your evaluation form, with any changes or comments suggested by your evaluator and instructor, in your employment portfolio for future reference.

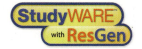

### StudyWARE™ Connection

Go to your software and view Carl, Dan, and Robin's videos, then give your feedback to decide how well each applicant prepared for their health care interview.

### In this step you will find

- a general description of a health care interview.
- "do's and don'ts" for health care interviews.
- a case study of a model health care interview.
- an activity with questions about the model health care interview.

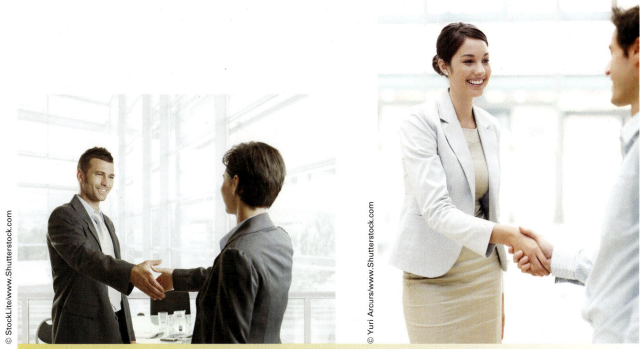

First impressions are important. You should look the interviewer in the eye, shake hands firmly, and smile.

## The Health Care Interview

The interview is your chance to sell yourself. You must give the impression that you have the skills necessary for the health care job you are seeking, that you are dependable, and that you get along well with people. Knowing what to do and what not to do during the interview ensures confidence and success. Be aware that most health care interviews usually contain the following four stages:

1. Introduction (what the health care position is about)
2. Questions about you and your qualifications
3. Questions from you about the job, health care facility, etc.
4. Closing remarks

**Stage 1: Introduction.** Start your interview like a winner. Show your enthusiasm. Your first greeting to the interviewer is critical to your being hired. Frequently interviewers make hiring decisions based on first impressions. Project confidence. Make a positive first impression by smiling and establishing eye contact with the interviewer when you introduce yourself. Smile, extend a firm handshake, and with a strong voice say, "Hello, Mrs. Sutton, I am Nancy Karr." Practice this technique speaking in front of a mirror, or with a family member or friend.

**Stage 2: Questions about you.** During the question stage, the employer will be leading the interview. The interviewer will be asking questions such as, "How would you describe your ability to work as a member of a health care team?" or "Why do you want to work for this health care facility?" Listen carefully. Answer all questions in a brief, concise manner. Relate all answers directly to skills you bring to the job. Relate your answers to the job description. Use standard English and avoid using slang. Two little magic words are "yes" and "no." Never respond "yeah" and "nah." Many interviewers believe that the best predictor of future performance is past performance. Therefore, they will ask for details on your experience. Be prepared to give specific examples of past performance.

**Stage 3: Questions from you.** This is the time when questions from you are welcomed.

Be sure to ask questions about the job and the health care facility. Not asking questions will make you appear unprepared. Have one or two thoughtfully prepared questions ready to refer to when asked. Review Step 5 for questions to ask. Employers are generally impressed when an applicant has good questions prepared in advance. Also remember that when you listen carefully to what is said during the interview, you may be able to follow up with a related question. Impress upon the interviewer that you would very much like to work for the health care facility.

**Stage 4: Closing remarks.** Watch for clues that indicate the interview is ending. Do not draw out the interview. If you are not immediately offered the job, you need to know when and how to follow up. To find out, you may ask a few final questions about the next step in the hiring process:

- Find out the date when the interviews will be completed. "When will the interviews be completed so I can follow up?"

- Find out how to contact the employer for the hiring decision. "Do you want me to call or e-mail you for the hiring decision?"

- Ask the interviewer for a business card. "May I have your business card?"

Instead of having you follow up, the employer may have a policy of contacting you. You still must send a thank-you letter, or note card, or both.

You will have one final moment to sell yourself. Show that you are interested in the job by *one* of the following:

- Stressing a strength. "I really care about the patients and pride myself on having a positive manner dealing with them."

- Stressing your willingness to learn. "I find learning new job responsibilities exciting."

- Mentioning a quality that was not discussed. "In addition to providing clinical services, my ability to provide preventive care education is important for the job of dental hygienist."

- Making a complimentary observation about the health care facility. "I am impressed about your organization's standards in patient care."

Smile, shake the interviewer's hand, and make your closing remark. Say, "I'm happy to have interviewed with you. Thank you for your time." This will leave a positive image.

# Do's and Don'ts When Interviewing

Study the list provided in Figure 1.6.1. Make a note of the items that you need to practice or review before your interview.

**FIGURE 1.6.1** Do's And Don'ts When Interviewing

**Do:**
- Shake the interviewer's hand firmly when introduced.
- Be courteous. Say, "Good morning, Miss Kinoshita. I am John Stevens."
- Know the interviewer's name in advance; use the name in conversation with the interviewer.
- Remain standing until you are asked to sit down.
- Make yourself comfortable and maintain your poise.
- Present your resume to the interviewer. Leave it with him or her.
- Allow the interviewer to lead the interview.
- Look the interviewer in the eye.
- Answer all questions directly and truthfully.
- Use correct English. Avoid slang.
- Be agreeable at all times.
- Demonstrate your ability to take constructive criticism in a mature way.
- Show interest in the health care facility.
- Ask questions about the job opening and the health care facility.
- Make the interviewer aware of your goals and your sincerity about planning your health care career.
- Indicate a willingness to start at the bottom. Do not expect too much too soon.
- Express your appreciation for the interviewer's time.
- Take any examination requested.

**Don't:**
- Place your handbag, briefcase, or other articles on the interviewer's desk. (Keep them in your hands or place them on the floor beside you.)
- Slouch in your chair.
- Play with your tie, rings, bracelets, hair, etc.
- Chew gum.
- Smoke.
- Make excuses, be evasive, hedge on facts presented in your record.
- Answer a question before the question is completely asked.
- Interrupt the interviewer.
- Brag.
- Mumble.
- Make jokes or argue.
- Gossip or bad-mouth former employers.
- Ask too many questions.
- Beg for work.

# A Model Interview

Carefully read the interview between Mr. Kevin Mansell, Human Resource Director, Danville Health Center, and job applicant Ms. Jessica Lee. This is a model interview. It is an ideal health care interview. Not all interviews are this smooth and perfect! The annotations highlight important benchmarks that occur in most interviews. Benchmarks are key points on which employers place special emphasis. As you read this model interview, think about how you can incorporate these

## ★ ★ MEDICAL TRANSCRIPTIONIST ★ ★
## DIAGNOSTIC IMAGING

Excellent Career Opportunity with Danville Health Center in CA. Seeking qualified candidates to transcribe medical dictation such as X-ray reports, operative procedures, autopsies, pathology reports, medical histories, discharge summaries, and special clinical notes. Requirements: completion of a medical transcriber vocational training program or 6 mos. experience as a medical transcriber in hospital, medical institution, or professional medical transcription services may be substituted for the required vocational training. Some additional training available for qualified candidate. Several positions available, permanent and temporary. Vacation, sick leave, and holiday coverage. Send resume to Kevin Mansell, Human Resource Director, Danville Health Center, 1793 California Dr., Alamo, CA 94507-2407, or fax to (925) 555-8700.

### Danville Health Center

An Equal Opportunity Employer

© Cengage Learning 2013

points in your own health care interviews. You can observe and learn good interview skills by the way Jessica conducts herself in the interview. Note that Jessica:

- Handles all aspects of the interview in a courteous manner.
- Takes an active role.
- Speaks with confidence and her confident attitude shows that she has done her homework.
- Describes her work skills well.
- Reflects research of the health care facility.
- Asks good questions.
- Is enthusiastic about the health care job.
- Is not passive.

Jessica speaks well and demonstrates she is a good prospect for employment. Jessica's assertive role offers pointers that can be used in your interviews.

Ms. Jessica Lee is seeking a medical record transcriptionist position that Danville Health Center has advertised in the newspaper ad, Figure 1.6.2. Jessica has sent in her application, resume, and cover letter, and has been granted an interview. Jessica walks into the Human Resource office of Mr. Kevin Mansell, the interviewer.

### Mr. Mansell:

Hello, Jessica, I'm Mr. Mansell. Please be seated.

### Jessica:

Thank you, Mr. Mansell. I am happy to meet you.

### Mr. Mansell:

Welcome to Danville Health Center, Jessica. Did you have any trouble finding the center?

*Get off to a good start.*

**Jessica:**

No, last week I programmed the address in my cell phone GPS, and I located your health care facility by driving here.

**Mr. Mansell:**

That shows good planning on your part, Jessica. According to your application and resume, you are interested in our medical record transcriptionist opening. Is that correct?

**Jessica:**

Yes, Mr. Mansell, I'd like to start my career in health care as a medical transcriptionist in a physician's medical center. I find such work challenging and rewarding.

**Mr. Mansell:**

Well, the job opening we have is in our medical records department. Your application indicates that you are a student taking intern training in medical transcription. Can you tell me more about your intern experience?

**Jessica:**

I am now working as an intern at Crestwood Hospital, where I've transcribed a variety of physician dictation, including initial patient office evaluations, exams and progress notes, and physician letters. My mentor has been satisfied with my progress in accurately understanding medical terminology. I have gained mastery over what I hear and what I key. I'm most proud of my correct punctuation, grammar, and spelling. Since starting my internship I have completed one patient file. I feel confident that I can apply all of this real work experience to Danville's medical records department.

**Mr. Mansell:**

You're right. We need someone who has the skills that you have described. You will soon graduate from New York Medical Community College as a medical transcriptionist. How do you think your education has helped prepare you for this position?

**Jessica:**

Many of the same secretarial skills I have developed in high school, and at New York Medical Community College are used in transcribing these medical reports. In high school I enjoyed my keying, science, English, and drama classes. At New York Medical Community College I earned excellent grades in anatomy, physiology, medical transcription, medical terminology, and medical office software. My keying speed is 70 words per minute with high accuracy. In addition, my high school oral communication and drama classes helped me to gain confidence when speaking to medical staff during my internship. I think I have developed skills from these courses that can be applied to the position of medical transcriptionist.

**Mr. Mansell:**

Yes, we need people with the right transcription and communication skills. If you were considered for this job opening, why would you want to work for Danville Health Center?

**Jessica:**

Well, there is a branch of Danville Health Center located where I live, and I have come to depend on it for my health care needs. I find your branch health center convenient, cost effective, and efficient. In fact, many of my friends are with companies that subscribe to your health services for some of the same reasons.

I also did some research on large medical facilities. I discovered that Danville Health Center was one of the leaders in the field. It has an excellent reputation for quality service. I would very much like to work for a health center with this kind of reputation.

Your center's website shows you are expanding statewide. This probably means that there will be opportunities for career development.

### Mr. Mansell:

Jessica, it's nice to know you are familiar with Danville Health Center's services and its reputation. With the opening of the new center—which has the job opening for which you applied—Danville Health Center plans to enlarge its network of health centers throughout the state. I think there will be many opportunities for career development. We have just designed a new career management-training program which should accommodate our expansion. We will need more management people as our health care centers open.

Jessica, this job is a standard 40-hour week, but we are looking for a person who can be on call for weekend work. Of course, when this is required, you would have an equal number of weekdays off. Would this be satisfactory for you?

### Jessica:

Working weekends would be fine. At Crestwood Hospital I work every Saturday. It seems to me having weekdays off could be an advantage. Which days would I have off if I were to work weekends?

### Mr. Mansell:

You probably would have Mondays and Tuesdays off. The final decision will depend upon the needs of our medical transcription department.

### Jessica:

That would be fine with me.

### Mr. Mansell:

Will our new Danville Health Center be a convenient work location?

### Jessica:

The location of the new center would work out fine for me. I recently purchased a car and should have no problem.

### Mr. Mansell:

Jessica, I see by your employment application you are presently working part-time for Hammond's Discount Bookstore. What did you like about working for Hammond's?

### Jessica:

Mr. Mansell, for the past two years I have been employed part-time at Hammond's while attending high school and New York Medical Community College. My part-time job has helped me pay for my education.

I've had a chance to develop effective communication skills interacting with customers, fellow associates, and store management. I sometimes work with a team but also complete job duties on my own. Hammond's is a fast-paced bookstore. On a typical workday time goes fast. I like having multiple tasks to do, such as assisting with counter sales and Web orders, organizing book stock and the cashier

*Note how Jessica's research makes a good impression.*

*Show you have a flexible attitude.*

stations, and assisting in creating store book displays. This helped me learn to organize my time and set priorities. Some of the skills that I have learned at Hammond's can be used in medical transcription work.

### Mr. Mansell:

Jessica, can you describe a stressful situation and how you handled it?

### Jessica:

Once during the Christmas season at Hammond's I agreed to work overtime but was still able to keep up with classes and homework. It helps that I am task oriented and self-motivated. I like to have a lot of work to do and see it get done. It's like I am competing with myself. It's like in medical transcription, "how many lines can I get done today."

**Be prepared to show a reference list/reference letters.**

### Mr. Mansell:

It's good to see a heavy workload poses little threat to you because transcription work sometimes has demanding time pressures. Jessica, do you have a reference list?

### Jessica:

Yes, I do. Here it is. (Hands Mr. Mansell her reference list.) Mr. Anderson at New York Medical Community College would be a good person to talk to about my transcription skills. He can be contacted before 10 a.m. weekdays.

### Mr. Mansell:

Jessica, do you have any questions you would like to ask?

**Be prepared to ask good questions.**

### Jessica:

Yes, can you give me more information about Danville's beginning employee training program and evaluation policy?

### Mr. Mansell:

All beginning employees start their training with a three-day welcome and orientation session. This covers our general operation and policies. After orientation, an employee is assigned to a department within the center. There the starting employee receives on-the-job training.

After this training period, as a new employee, you are placed on probation for six months. Every two months during this probationary period, your supervisor will evaluate you. After successfully completing the probationary period, you would be classified as a "regular" employee and receive a raise in pay.

Each regular employee is evaluated twice a year, generally every six months. After each successful evaluation, the employee earns a raise in pay. Our employee benefit package is standard for this industry. Danville gives employees holiday pay and two weeks of vacation after one year of service. We also provide medical and dental insurance coverage and have a 401(k) retirement plan. Does that sufficiently explain what you wanted to know in these areas?

### Jessica:

Yes, thank you. That gives me some good information.

### Mr. Mansell:

We haven't discussed wages. What pay do you expect?

### Jessica:

Could you tell me what the pay range is for a beginning medical transcriptionist at Danville Health Center?

**Mr. Mansell:**

Our pay range varies, depending on the department. For example, in our medical records department, the starting salary is $600.00 a week. After this, your pay is based on longevity and ability. Your supervisor will judge your ability level according to department standards. When your new employee orientation is scheduled, you will be given further details about this department wage and ability standard. How does that sound to you?

**Jessica:**

That sounds very good.

**Mr. Mansell:**

When could you start work if hired?

**Jessica:**

I would have to give my Hammond's manager, Mr. Sayers, notice that I will be leaving. I could start in two weeks, immediately after graduation from New York Medical Community College. When do you expect to complete interviewing for this position, Mr. Mansell?

**Mr. Mansell:**

I still have a few people left to interview, but I hope to finish by next Tuesday.

**Jessica:**

May I call you Wednesday morning? I am very interested in working for Danville Health Center. You have convinced me that Danville Health Center would make an excellent employer. May I have your business card?

**Mr. Mansell:**

Certainly. (Hands Jessica his business card.) We would like you to follow up!

**Jessica:**

Thank you for this opportunity, Mr. Mansell. Now that my interview is over, I am even more convinced that Danville is the health center for me. I really am impressed with its career possibilities. It was good talking with you.

**Mr. Mansell:**

You are welcome, Jessica. Thank you for interviewing with Danville Health Center. Good-bye.

*Jessica does a great job. She does not ask for a specific pay rate.*

*Establish a follow-up phone call; ask for a business card.*

*Leave in a courteous and positive way.*

*Don't forget a post-interview thank-you letter.*

## Activity 10

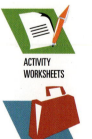

ACTIVITY
WORKSHEETS

PORTFOLIO
UPDATE

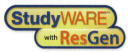

### Health Care Case Study Questions

When you have finished reading the interview, remove Activity 10 in Section 3, and answer the case questions. By answering these questions, you will learn important interviewing skills. When you have completed this activity to your satisfaction, show it to your instructor for evaluation. Then place it in your employment portfolio for future health care interview preparation.

### StudyWARE™ Connection

Go to your software and view Carl and Dan's participant perspectives and Robin's video and review the importance of first impressions and listening in a health care interview.

### In this step you will find

- how to follow up a health care job interview with a letter.

- a sample health care post-interview letter, post-interview note, and follow-up e-mail.

- an activity to construct a health care post-interview letter.

- how to evaluate a health care job offer.

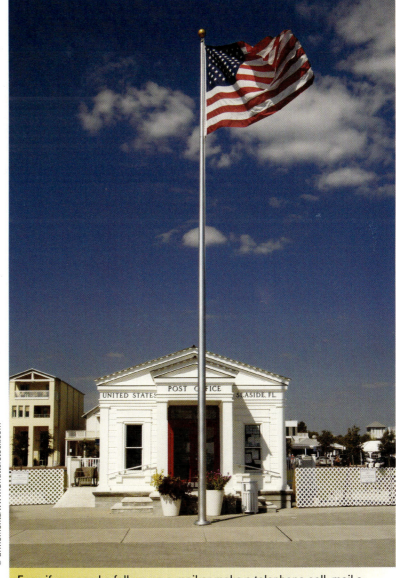

© urmoments/www.Shutterstock.com

Even if you send a follow-up e-mail or make a telephone call, mail a thank-you letter within 24 hours.

# How to Follow Up a Health Care Job Interview with a Letter

After all interviews for a health care position have been completed, there sometimes may be two or three equally qualified applicants for the one job opening. All of the applicants would probably make good employees, but only one may be selected. However, one determining factor in making such a selection may be based on the applicant who exhibits the strongest desire for or interest in the job. Therefore, the applicant who follows up on the interview with a thank-you letter may be the one selected for the job.

If you really want a particular health care job, write a letter immediately after the interview and mail it within 24 hours. Do not put this off! A post-interview letter makes a powerful impression. It shows you are really interested in the job. An employer may consider you a better candidate because of the letter you have written. Pay as much attention to the quality and accuracy of this letter as to your earlier correspondence. Proofread your letter before you mail it. If you have an error on this follow-up letter, you could lose your chance at a job you want. See Figure 1.7.1 for a sample post-interview letter. Read it carefully.

Use the following guidelines when writing a post-interview letter:

1. Address your letter to the person who interviewed you. (You should have the interviewer's business card for the information you need.)

2. Thank the potential employer, and state the position for which you are applying. Restate your interest in the position and/or the health care facility.

3. Briefly restate those qualifications that make you well suited for the job.

4. Add any additional information you failed to mention in the interview.

5. Include a date when you will follow up with the interviewer, and indicate how you will do so (e.g., phone call or e-mail).

An alternative to a keyed letter is a handwritten note. Send a handwritten note only if your handwriting is legible. A handwritten thank-you note is a shortened version of a follow-up letter. Use plain, good-quality note cards and avoid colored stationery because it does not look professional. Figure 1.7.2 shows a sample handwritten note.

# How to Follow Up a Health Care Interview for a Hiring Decision

How to find out if a hiring decision has been made depends on the arrangements you have made in the interview and what the interviewer would like you to do. You must ask in the interview how you should follow up. The interviewer may want you to phone on a particular date after the interviews are completed, or e-mail the facility for the hiring decision. By making a prearranged phone call, you can determine if a decision has been made and restate your interest in the position and in working for the health care facility. Here is a four-step follow-up plan when you call a health care facility.

1. **Reintroduce yourself and restate your interest in the job.** "Hello, Mrs. Vaughn. My name is Miguel Nieves. I interviewed with you last Wednesday for the job of Dental Assistant. I wanted to thank you for discussing the position and let you know again that I am very much interested in the job."

**FIGURE 1.7.1** Post-Interview Letter

1″ (Line 7)

**AMY FRUHWIRTH**

3841 Geneva St., Baltimore, MD 21218 (410) 555-8824 Cell (410) 555-6329
afruhwirth@gmail.com
2-4S

1″

September 15, 20—

4S

Mrs. Susan King
Office Manager
Fremont Hospital
3877 Erie Street
Baltimore, MD 21218
2S

Dear Mrs. King
2S

**A** Thank you for giving me the opportunity to interview for the position of Medical
Secretary with your hospital. The interview was interesting as well as informative.
2S

**B** The interview confirmed my opinion that I have the skills required for the Medical
Secretary position with your hospital. My knowledge of medical terminology, anatomy,
physiology, keying, word processing, telephone techniques, and transcription would
be beneficial to Fremont Hospital.
2S

1″

**C** I am very interested in working for Fremont Hospital as a Medical Secretary. I believe
this position would provide a challenging career opportunity for me in my chosen
field. If hired, I would prove to be a most productive and dependable employee.
I will call you on September 21st as agreed in our interview.
2S

Sincerely

*Amy Fruhwirth*   4S

Amy Fruhwirth

| | |
|---|---|
| **A** | Thank-you and positive comment about interview |
| **B** | Emphasize strengths |
| **C** | Continued interest and additional reasons for hiring |

**FIGURE 1.7.2**  Post-Interview Note

January 8, 20—

Dear Mr. Jung:

Thank you for the informative physical therapy assistant interview yesterday. You were kind to point out the new ultrasound and electrical stimulation treatment programs.

I would very much enjoy being able to assist with exercise treatments in such an innovative environment. My clinical experience gives me confidence for Redwood's Physical Therapy procedures.

Thank you for your time and consideration.

Sincerely,

**Sherry Louie**

(845) 555-4572
slouie@yahoo.com

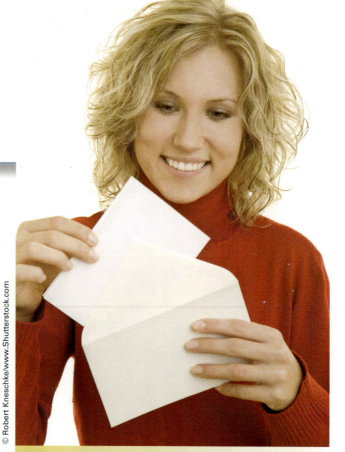

Make your thank-you personal with a handwritten note.

© Robert Kneschke/www.Shutterstock.com

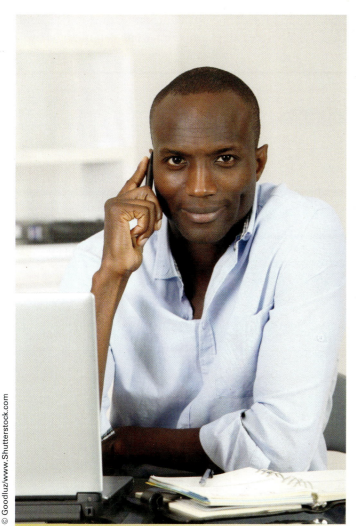

Make a prearranged phone call to find out if a hiring decision has been made.

**2.** **Find out if a hiring decision has been made.** "Has a hiring decision been made for the position of Dental Assistant?"

If you are offered the job, express your thanks and ask for the starting date so you can make resignation arrangements with your current employer. However, if a decision has been made and you did *not* get the job, ask the interviewer how you might have been a more competitive candidate. You could say the following:

"I am sorry you don't feel I am the person for the job. At some future date I would like to interview again with your dental clinic. Could you give me some suggestions for being a stronger and more qualified candidate?"

Or you might say the following:

"Thank you for considering me for this position. I would appreciate your comments on my resume and interviewing skills."

You may receive constructive criticism that will help you in future interviews. Make this a learning experience. Keep in mind, however, that health care facilities are not obligated to answer your question.

**3.** **If a hiring decision has *not* been made, add any additional thoughts you may not have covered when you interviewed.** "I did not mention in our interview my present plans for enrolling in a dental accounting class to learn Intuit software. Having some dental accounting training would be helpful when taking inventory—ordering and monitoring dental supplies and equipment in a dental clinic."

Emphasize once again your strengths for the job:

"Mrs. Vaughn, the interview confirmed my belief that I have the skills required for the position of Dental Assistant. My experience in dealing with people and my attention to detail are valuable skills that will be needed for this job. I also believe that the position of Dental Assistant will be a challenging career opportunity."

**4.** **Thank the interviewer.** "Thank you for your time. When may I call you for a decision?"

If you did not get the job, thank the interviewer again for considering you for the position, as well as any feedback he or she may have given you about your resume or interviewing skills.

At the end of the interview, you may find that the employer would like you to follow up for a hiring decision by e-mail rather than by phone. If that is the case, be sure to use your professional e-mail and include the date of the interview, job title, and your contact information. In the subject line put your name, the job title, and the word "interview." Figure 1.7.3 provides an example of what you might write in a follow-up e-mail.

---

**FIGURE 1.7.3** Post-Interview E-mail

June 2, 20—

Dear Mr. Morimoto:

Thank you for interviewing me June 1st for the surgical technologist position. I enjoyed meeting you and appreciate learning more about Glenville Hospital.

I am excited about the possibility of joining your team. If hired, I would be a dependable employee.

No matter how many people you interview, you won't find anyone who wants to work for you more than I do. I will call for a hiring decision on June 9 as agreed upon in our interview.

Sincerely,

*David Greenstein*

(925) 555-1472
dgreenstein@gmail.com

---

# Activity 11

ACTIVITY
WORKSHEETS

PORTFOLIO
UPDATE

## Preparing a Health Care Post-Interview Letter

Based on the information in the following scenario, remove Activity 11 in Section 3, and draft a post-interview letter. Refer to the sample letter, Figure 1.7.1, to write your health care post-interview letter. After you have drafted your letter, show it to your instructor for evaluation. Make any necessary corrections. Key and save your letter on the same thumb drive that has your resume and other material from this manual. Print your final post-interview letter on the same quality paper used for your resume. Place your printed post-interview letter in your employment portfolio for future reference.

### Scenario for Activity 11

You have interviewed for the health care job of (insert your job choice). The job pays well. The working conditions and hours meet your needs, and you are a good prospect for this position. Mr. David Souza, the personnel manager, has told you that he has other applicants to interview. You have decided to follow up immediately with a post-interview letter and later with a prearranged phone call to Mr. Souza. His employment address is St. Louis Medical/Dental Clinic, 200 Washington Avenue, St. Louis, MO 63103. You may use a health care facility of your choice if you prefer. Use the Internet and search for hospitals or health care facilities in your area, or use your local newspaper's employment section list of other health care facilities and positions for this post-interview letter.

# Evaluating a Health Care Job Offer

Congratulations! Your hard work has paid off. You are offered the health care job. Now you will have to decide whether or not to accept it. This decision should be an easy one to make if you have gathered the necessary information about the health care facility and the position, and if you have evaluated the job's advantages and disadvantages.

The information you have gathered, along with the following questions, will help you make the right decision.

1. Does this health care position provide the kind of work that will be satisfying day after day?

2. Can you live on the wages being offered?

3. How are wage increases earned?

4. Does the health care facility offer satisfactory job security? (Job security is how the health care facility deals with layoffs and other unemployment issues.)

5. Is the health care facility's benefit package satisfactory?

6. Is your supervisor the kind of person for whom you could easily work?

7. Are the co-workers the kind of people with whom you could easily work?

8. Is the health care facility location convenient?

9. Does this health care job offer opportunities for training, education, and advancement?

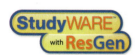

## StudyWARE™ Connection

Go to your software and watch Robin's participant perspective and summaries for Carol, Dan, and Robin, then supply your feedback for after their health care interviews.

### In this step you will find

- how to start a new health care job.

- a procedure for acing your performance review.

- how your positive personal qualities count.

- an activity to identify health care personal qualities.

- advice that can help you grow in your health care job.

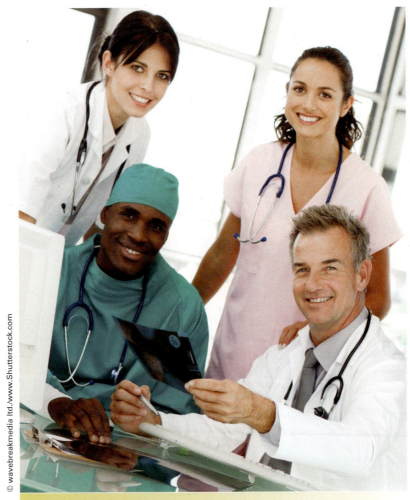

© wavebreakmedia ltd./www.Shutterstock.com

Be positive. Work with a smile.

# Starting a Health Care Job

You have accepted the health care job offer! This is your dream job. Now send a note to all of the people who have helped you, relaying the good news. You will find success comes easily in your new job if you get off to a good start. Be assured your demeanor and actions will be scrutinized during the first days and weeks you are working. This is a time during which your professional personality and work attitude should shine. First impressions are often lasting impressions, so be immaculate in your appearance. Give serious thought to how you want to be perceived by your health care co-workers and supervisor after several months have passed. Next, make an intentional effort to develop and/or improve the goals shown here. Ask yourself how committed you are to reaching each of them. Be determined to build your professional image. Always keep in mind the quality of your service directly or indirectly affects the patient outcomes. These guidelines will help ensure a successful start in your new health care job. Review this list before work each day and hold yourself accountable.

- **Be positive.** Work with a smile. Show your enthusiasm for your job responsibilities. Pay attention to the ways things are done, then adjust and be eager to learn. Take responsibility for any mistakes and correct your errors. Give thought to how you are going to avoid repeating them.

- **Intentionally plan your job growth.** Get to know the employee handbook. Find out if there are any unwritten policies. Review your job description. Learn the priorities of your supervisor. Pay close attention and take notes during your new employee orientation. Join the professional health care association specific to your job and attend meetings. Attend other events your health care facility offers.

- **Be accountable.** Arrive to work early. Do not miss a day of work or ask for a day off. Complete your job duties on time and be punctual to meetings.

- **Be a team member.** Do not hang back when you have the opportunity to join a group effort. Show your support and offer to help. Be sure to show your appreciation for any help given as you learn your job duties.

- **Be a trusted professional.** Make a list of the names of the co-workers you meet to help get to know them. Be friendly with all the people with whom you work as well as the people above you. But, "fitting in" does not mean joining in "office politics." Your job future depends on your loyalty, confidentiality, and ability to cooperate with everyone. Look for a successful health care professional who could be your mentor and guide your health care career.

- **Listen more than you talk.** Make it a high priority to focus on what is said when you are listening. Intentionally think about what you say before you say it. Do not be afraid to ask questions to make sure you understand and are following the correct procedures. By doing this you may be able to clear up possible misunderstandings. Make a deliberate effort to stop and think before acting when a problem arises. Your focus and judgment may result in an effective solution.

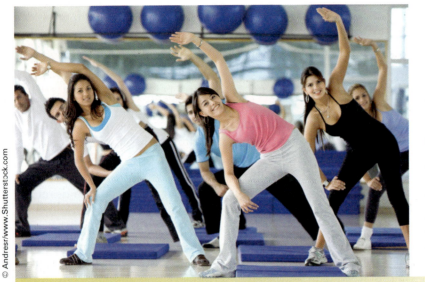

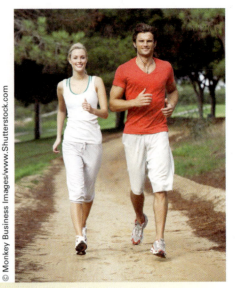

Take care of yourself. Be proactive about your health.

- **Practice healthy living.** When you are at your personal best, everyone benefits. Good personal hygiene and grooming are mandatory for working in a health care facility. Be proactive about your health. Get enough sleep, good nutrition, and exercise to have enough stamina to cope with the stress of your job.

As you start your new health care job, these goals will give you greater direction and focus. They are the foundation you need to be at your professional best.

# Ace Your Performance Review

One way you can make the most of your health care job is by having a good performance review. Most likely you will have formal performance reviews with your supervisor on a scheduled basis. These job evaluations are designed to help you improve your performance, determine if you will keep your health care job, and get a raise in pay and/or a promotion. Your health care job description tells you most—but not all—that is expected of you on the job. Your supervisor may not take time to spell out some of what you are expected to know—and what you do not know may cause problems for you in your job. You should have a clear picture of what is expected of you before your formal performance review so you can perform your best and get a good job evaluation.

Here are steps to take before your formal performance review with your supervisor. Your goal is to have job expectation transparency. This means that you and your supervisor should agree on your job expectations. These steps will help clear up any potential misunderstandings. They will help put you in control of your job.

1. **Do a self-assessment of how well you perform your health care job duties.**
   Take an objective look at your job performance. Make sure you are performing all of your job duties to the best of your abilities. Review your job

description, if you have one, and make a list of the job duties. If you do not have a job description, make a list of the exact job duties that you have been assigned. Evaluate yourself honestly. If you find any deficiencies, begin to make corrections.

2. **Talk to your supervisor about what is expected of you.** Ask for a casual time that is private and convenient for your supervisor to meet with you. Give a copy of your duties to your supervisor for a review. Tell your supervisor that you would like to make sure your list of job duties is complete, and that you would appreciate any suggestions. Be sure to ask your supervisor which personal work qualities he or she feels are most important, and which you may need to improve. Make note of any suggestions from your supervisor. For example, your supervisor may value initiative, teamwork, diversity, and continuous improvement. You should leave this meeting with a clear understanding of what is expected of you. Knowing your job duties and personal qualities will help you become a more confident and productive worker.

3. **Do a daily self-check.** Each day until the date of your performance review, check yourself against the health care job duties and personal work qualities that you listed. Record any dates you went beyond your regular duties, and make a note of your accomplishments, such as the following:

   - Working overtime to cover for a health care employee who was ill.

   - Reporting early to help handle a special health care team project.

   - Taking a class, or attending a seminar or conference to improve your health care job knowledge and skills.

## Your Health Care Performance Review

Now you can be confident and go to your health care performance review with energy and enthusiasm. Be prepared to discuss your strengths. Have a copy of your job duties and accomplishments with dates and notes of how you went beyond your normal responsibilities. Your supervisor may not be aware of some of the additional tasks you performed. Confidently accept responsibility for any areas your supervisor says you could improve. Ask for specific suggestions of what you can do to improve in these areas. Share with your supervisor what you would like to achieve in the future. Show you are confident, and be determined to contribute by finding ways to be of value to the health care facility. Keeping your supervisor informed about your progress, combined with your own self-evaluation, can help you reach your full potential within the health care facility.

# Positive Personal Qualities Count

Your personality is made up of a variety of personal qualities, such as how you get along with other people, how you handle pressure, and how you accept responsibility. These are important qualities a health care worker must have to be effective. Your personality affects your attitude, the decisions you make, and your performance. If your health care job complements your personality, you will usually be happy with your work. Personal qualities are often as important to your health care job success as previous work experience and academic qualifications. Interpersonal and communication skills are needed to interact well in a variety of health care situations. From working with your health care co-worker team members to the relationship with your supervisor and patients, good personal qualities are paramount. There are many positive personal qualities that can help you succeed in your health care job.

In Step 4 you researched a particular health care job using the O*Net OnLine website. You found the "Work Styles" category and highlighted just one personal quality that you found important to you in your chosen health care job. Yet there were many personal qualities that were identified as needed in your health care job.

For example, if you research Licensed Practical and Licensed Vocational Nurses, you can see the following personal qualities described under the category "Work Styles":

**Dependability**—Job requires being reliable, responsible, and dependable, and fulfilling obligations.

**Integrity**—Job requires being honest and ethical.

**Attention to Detail**—Job requires being careful about detail and thorough in completing work tasks.

**Concern for Others**—Job requires being sensitive to others' needs and feelings and being understanding and helpful on the job.

**Self-Control**—Job requires maintaining composure, keeping emotions in check, controlling anger, and avoiding aggressive behavior, even in very difficult situations.

**Cooperation**—Job requires being pleasant with others on the job and displaying a good-natured, cooperative attitude.

**Social Orientation**—Job requires preferring to work with others rather than alone, and being personally connected with others on the job.

**Stress Tolerance**—Job requires accepting criticism and dealing calmly and effectively with high-stress situations.

**Initiative**—Job requires a willingness to take on responsibilities and challenges.

**Independence**—Job requires developing one's own ways of doing things, guiding oneself with little or no supervision, and depending on oneself to get things done.

All health care jobs listed in the O*Net OnLine website have a "Work Styles" category. Now that you are starting your health care job, become familiar with **all** of the personal qualities described for your job. By concentrating on them you will develop your unique professional competence.

**ACTIVITY WORKSHEETS**

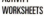

**WEBSITE**

**PORTFOLIO UPDATE**

## Identifying Health Care Personal Qualities

You will need a copy of your job title information from O*Net OnLine to complete this activity. You may use a copy you made of your job title from the research you did on O*Net in Step 4 and placed in your employment portfolio. Otherwise, go online to the O*Net OnLine.org home page and select "Find Occupations." Key in your job title and you will be linked to detailed information about it. Make a copy of your job title information. Using your printed copy, find the category "Work Styles" and read the headings followed by a description of the personal qualities that are needed for your health care job.

Next, remove Activity 12 in Section 3 and follow the directions for completing this activity. When you have completed the activity to your satisfaction, show it to your instructor for evaluation. Then place it and the copy of your O*Net job description in your employment portfolio as a resource for your health care job.

## Continue to Grow in Your Health Care Job

Many health care jobs are stressful, due in part to the physical and emotional demands. In order to function at your best, there are ways to manage your stress. Along with maintaining a good performance review, as time goes on, there are other ways you can improve your health care job satisfaction. Some aspects of your health care job, such as management, including company policies, will not be within your power to change. Accept these realities. Keep in mind your overall feelings about your job and do not dwell on something you cannot control. Concentrate on changes you can make. By taking control, you will improve your physical and mental health and have a better relationship with your co-workers, supervisor, and patients. Practice using your sense of humor to relieve stress, tension, or anxiety. Laughter used appropriately with your co-workers, or even with patients, can have psychological and physical benefits. If you improve some health care work skill or personal work quality, you may find that other parts of your job that once seemed discouraging will not bother you anymore. If you ace your performance review, develop the personal qualities described for your job in your O*Net research in this step, and consider some of the following suggestions, you could very well be in line for a raise or promotion:

- Maintain a positive attitude.
- Develop a mentoring relationship.
- Join your professional organization.
- Keep a good balance between your health care employment and personal life.
- Continue your education and learn new skills to increase your value to your health care facility.
- Improve any human relations problems you have at your health care facility.
- Redesign your work.
- Be proactive about your health.

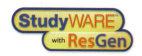

## StudyWARE™ Connection

Go to your software and quiz yourself on how to start a health care job.

# Leaving a Health Care Job . . . Gracefully

## Introduction

Section 2, Leaving a Health Care Job…Gracefully, contains Steps 1–3 with valuable advice and insight concerning how to leave a job in health care gracefully and with excellent references. There is far more to leaving a job than saying, "I quit."

### Step 1: Questions to Consider Before Leaving a Health Care Job

This step presents important questions you should ask yourself before leaving a health care job. A health care case study activity will help you decide how to make a job-leaving decision.

### Step 2: The Best Way to Leave a Health Care Job

This step explains the positive way to leave a health care job. You will learn the importance of following health care facility policy. Included is what to say to your employer and your co-workers, and how to write a resignation letter that could lead to a good recommendation.

### Step 3: Health Care Reference Letter

This step shows you how to obtain a reference letter that can be used to obtain future jobs. This section ends by outlining positive procedures for handling serious employment problems. If you are laid off, downsized, or fired, this information is essential.

### In this step you will find

- information on when to leave a health care job.
- questions to consider before leaving a health care job.
- a quiz to help you decide if you should leave a health care job.
- a health care case study activity.

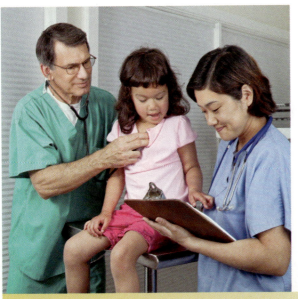 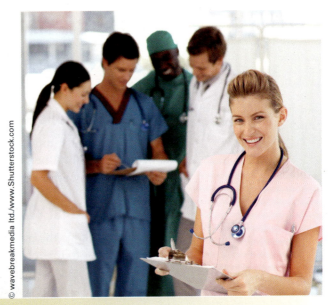

Consider all of the advantages and disadvantages of a health care job change.

## Why Does Someone Leave a Health Care Job?

Most people make many job changes during their working lives. People have many reasons for deciding to leave a health care employer. These include the following:

- Finding another health care job that shows more promise or pays better.
- No longer feeling satisfaction with the health care work.
- Being passed over for promotion.
- Wishing to make a health care career change.
- Having the job affect your health.
- Having important responsibilities taken away.

# Questions to Consider Before Leaving a Health Care Job

Choosing to leave a health care job can be a very emotional, stressful decision. It can cause insecurity and a loss of career progress. You should understand the impact of leaving a job and look for ways to improve your job before rashly deciding to quit. Carefully consider the following before you leave a job:

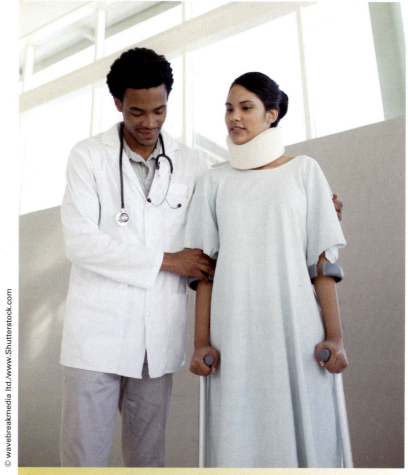

As you learn new skills you may be able to set new health care career goals.

1. **Job Satisfaction.** If your health care job is not satisfying or challenging, have you spoken to your supervisor about making changes? Have you looked into other jobs within your health care facility? Have you applied for additional training, education, or special health care programs? Are there any promotional opportunities available at your health care facility?

2. **Financial Impact.** What is the financial impact of your decision? At this time, can you afford to leave this health care job? Can you obtain a comparable health care job that will provide equal or higher pay and benefits? What benefits will you lose (medical, dental, etc.), and can you afford to lose them? Not all financial decisions are short term. What impact does leaving your health care employment have on long-term benefits such as retirement and employee profit-sharing plans?

3. **Personal Conflicts.** Have you started by examining yourself? Do you realize that you can only change yourself? Can you change your actions and reaction to the other person? Are you sure that the other person is really the problem, or are you overreacting? Have you done everything possible to resolve any personality conflict with your supervisor or co-worker? Have you discussed the conflict with your supervisor or co-worker with whom you are having the difficulty? Is it possible that this person will eventually be transferred out of your work area?

4. **Work Environment.** What is it about your environment that is not positive? An example of work environment includes having a comfortable and well-equipped workspace where health and safety standards are met. Is the environment conducive to patient satisfaction? Have you discussed ways to improve the work environment with your supervisor? Is it possible to transfer to another workstation within your health care facility?

5. **Career Plans.** What impact will leaving your health care job have on your career plans? If you are considering employment with another health care facility, what do you know about the facility's financial condition, goals and objectives, management philosophy, and competition? Have you compared the features of another health care facility with your present health care facility? Have you researched the demand for this job on O*Net OnLine?

To decide when it is time to leave, it may help to make a list of the advantages and disadvantages of your current health care employment situation, and you can take the quiz in Figure 2.1.1 to help you think through your decision.

---

**FIGURE 2.1.1** Ten-Question Quiz

### Is It Time for a Health Care Job Change?
### Ten Questions to Help You Decide

Whenever you are wondering if it is time to change a health care job, take the following ten-question quiz. Check ( ✔ ) a yes or no box for each question. When you have completed the quiz, add your yes and no answers. If you have answered **more** questions *yes* than *no*, you may be ready for a health care employment change.

Yes No

☐ ☐ 1. Does your health care manager ignore your suggestions?

☐ ☐ 2. Have you been passed over consistently for a promotion?

☐ ☐ 3. Do you feel underpaid for work you perform?

☐ ☐ 4. Is your health care employment harming your physical or emotional health?

☐ ☐ 5. Do you find yourself constantly watching the clock at work?

☐ ☐ 6. Are promises made to you by your health care employer but not kept?

☐ ☐ 7. Have you received poor performance evaluations?

☐ ☐ 8. Would your co-workers say you are a difficult person with whom to work?

☐ ☐ 9. Do you feel unrecognized for your good work?

☐ ☐ 10. Do you have more bad workdays than good?

## Trust Your Instincts

If you go through the suggestions in this step, you will know when it is right to leave a health care job. Respect your inner feelings regarding your employment. Since your health care job represents a large portion of your daily life, it is important to feel good about what you are doing. Regardless of your reason, never let leaving a health care job become a negative, stressful experience. If a paycheck is necessary, make sure you have another job (or at least the promise of one) before leaving your current job. You can use the employment information in Section 1 of this manual to find a health care job whether you are currently employed or not.

## Activity 13

**ACTIVITY WORKSHEETS**

**PORTFOLIO UPDATE**

### Health Care Case Study—Decision Time

Carefully read the case study about Aaron Rodgers in Section 3, Activity 13. Aaron needs your help to decide what to do about his health care job. Remove the activity worksheet provided, and create a list showing the advantages and disadvantages of Aaron remaining in his current employment. Decide for yourself what his decision should be. If you decide Aaron should remain, tell what he could do to improve his health care job situation. To help you determine what Aaron should do, be sure to review the questions and suggestions found in this step. When you have completed this activity to your satisfaction, show it to your instructor for evaluation and class discussion. Place it in your employment portfolio for future reference.

Now you know the questions to ask yourself, and a process to follow, before leaving a health care job. Refer to the information in this step when deciding if you should keep or leave a health care job in the future.

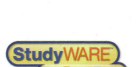

### StudyWARE™ Connection

Go to your software and view the photo gallery for this step for what to consider before leaving a job, then review the remaining photos for other helpful tips for your health care career.

**In this step you will find**

- positive ways to leave a health care job.
- what to tell your health care employer.
- what to tell your co-workers.
- a sample health care resignation letter.
- a health care resignation letter activity.
- a health care exit conversation activity.

## Positive Ways to Leave a Health Care Job

Your employer expects you to know how to end your health care employment in a positive, mature way. Do not feel you are doing the wrong thing by leaving your job. According to U.S. government statistics, the average person will have six or seven different jobs during a lifetime. Since your first job probably will not be your last, it is important to know how to leave a health care job in a positive way.

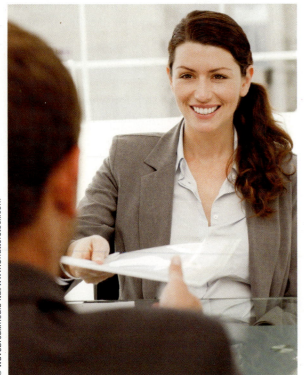

Present a resignation letter to your health care employer before you tell any co-workers.

© wavebreakmedia ltd./www.Shutterstock.com

Even when your work situation was not good, you must remember that leaving a health care job in a businesslike manner protects your reputation and may help you obtain a favorable reference. Keep the door open for a future career position you may want with your former health care employer. Perhaps one day you may even want to work with a former supervisor or co-worker at another health care facility.

### Follow Organization Policy

Usually two weeks notice is expected, although some health care employers may require more or less time in order to hire and train your replacement. Your health care employer will appreciate an offer to help train your replacement and will most likely remember your spirit of cooperation. This could definitely influence the type of reference you receive.

### Write a Health Care Resignation Letter

This letter informs your health care employer and/or supervisor of your decision to leave. Present this letter

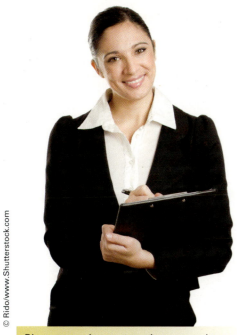

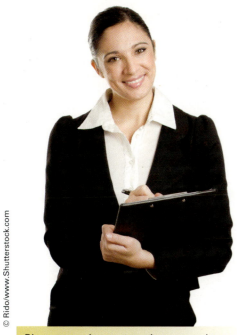
Plan your exit conversation so you leave your health care job on a positive note.

to your supervisor before telling your co-workers and friends that you are leaving. You do not want your employer to find out from another employee that you are leaving. A well-written health care resignation letter could lead to a good recommendation. Be sure to include the following required elements:

- The date you wish to leave your health care facility
- Your reason(s) for leaving a health care job (keep them positive)
- Your thanks for the professional development you have acquired
- Your appreciation of the health care organization and the people with whom you have worked

Figure 2.2.1 provides a good example of a well-written resignation letter. Study it carefully.

## The Exit Conversation: What to Tell Your Health Care Employer

Some large health care facilities have formal structured exit interviews for employees who have resigned. Many health care employers have a less formal policy for leaving, a simple exit conversation. The exit interview or conversation may be completed with your health care supervisor or with someone from the human relations department.

When you hand in your resignation letter, your supervisor will expect you to tell why you are leaving. Prepare a positive reason for leaving. You might say:

- "I have found a health care job with a shorter commute."
- "I have accepted an advanced health care position."
- "I have accepted a job in a larger health care facility."
- "I am making a health care career change that allows me to use my new skills."

Before you have your exit conversation, make a list of some positive things you have learned from your health care job. Think hard! Your experience may have taught you job skills such as computerized record-keeping, medical office bookkeeping, laboratory techniques, or safety precautions. Your job may have also improved such work habits as communicating well with team members, ability to meet deadlines, following policies and procedures, respecting diversity, supporting patients in a positive way, and learning coping skills to be able to work under stressful conditions.

**FIGURE 2.2.1** Resignation Letter

1" (Line 7)

**COLLEEN VINCENT**
2338 Galscow Road
Houston, TX 77057
(731) 555-2674

2–4S

1"

June 18, 20--

4S

Mr. John Sayers
Director of Personnel
Ford Medical Center
2450 High Street
Houston, TX 77057

2S

Dear Mr. Sayers

2S

**A** Please accept this letter as notice of my resignation to become effective July 1, 20--. I have accepted a position as a Medical Record Supervisor with the Stanford Medical Group of San Francisco. I am to report to work on July 14, 20--.

1"

2S

**B** I would like to thank Ford Medical Center for giving me the opportunity to learn new and useful medical office information procedures. Your on-the-job electronic health records (HER) and codifying training program was of great professional value.

2S

**C** It has been a pleasure to have worked for Ford Medical Center. I will always be proud of my association with such a fine health care organization and medical staff.

2S

Sincerely

*Colleen Vincent*      4S

Colleen Vincent

> **A** Date of resignation and positive reason(s) for leaving
>
> **B** Appreciation of professional development
>
> **C** Appreciation of fellow employees and health care facility

## Job Skills I Have Learned

_____

_____

_____

_____

## Work Habits I Have Improved

_____

_____

_____

_____

# A Model Health Care Exit Conversation

The following conversation is a good example of how to inform your health care employer that you are leaving your job. Note that Paul's exit conversation is short and to the point. He is polite and leaves a positive impression.

"Ms. Choi, it is necessary for me to give you and Seagate Medical Center notice that I am leaving. (Hands letter of resignation to Ms. Choi.) I have enjoyed working with the many great people that make up this health care facility. I have accepted a position with Kirkland Medical Group as Medical Records Supervisor. By making this change, I will be able to develop and improve my medical record knowledge and management skills.

I want to thank you for the excellent medical office administration experience I have gained working for Seagate Medical Center. I have learned the importance of sound health care organizational strategies and effective leadership skills.

Would you like me to train my replacement?"

# What to Tell Your Co-Workers

After you have told your health care employer that you are leaving and submitted your resignation letter, you may also want to tell your fellow employees. Keep your remarks short and your reasons for leaving positive. **Make sure your reasons for leaving are the same positive ones you expressed to management in your resignation letter and exit conversation.** Tell your fellow employees that it was great working with them and you will miss them. Whatever you do, do not brag about any greater benefits of your new job. Your co-workers may become jealous. Save those comments for your family and for close friends not associated with your health care facility. Out of fairness to your health care organization and co-workers, do not mention any negative conditions about the job you are leaving. This will reflect poorly on you. Your fellow workers will not appreciate negative remarks about their health care employer.

Activity 14

**ACTIVITY WORKSHEETS**

**PORTFOLIO UPDATE**

## Writing a Health Care Resignation Letter

Carefully read the sample health care resignation letter in this step. Remember a time that you left a job or assume that you are resigning from your present job, or one you have in mind for the future. Assume that you have been successful and learned a great deal. Using the sample health care resignation letter as a guide, write your own health care resignation letter. Remove the Activity 14 worksheet provided in Section 3. After you have drafted your letter, show it to your instructor for evaluation. Make any necessary corrections. Key your final health care resignation letter and save the file to the same thumb drive as your resume and other documents. Print your final resignation letter on the same size and quality paper used for your resume. Place a printed copy of your health care resignation letter in your employment portfolio for future reference.

Remember that when you leave a health care job, you should also update your resume with new skills that you have learned.

Activity 15

**ACTIVITY WORKSHEETS**

**PORTFOLIO UPDATE**

## Health Care Exit Conversation

Using Paul's model health care exit conversation in this step as a guide, write your own exit conversation. Address your conversation to either a present or a past employer. If you have never held a job, select a health care employer that you have researched. Remember to be discreet, and keep your exit conversation short and to the point. Remove the paper provided for Activity 15 in Section 3, and write your exit conversation. After you have written your health care exit conversation, show it to your instructor for evaluation. Make any necessary corrections. Place your completed exit conversation in your employment portfolio for future reference.

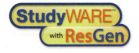

## StudyWARE™ Connection

Go to your software and complete the assessment activity relating to the best way to leave a health care job.

**In this step you will find**

- the definition of a health care reference letter.
- how to obtain a health care reference letter.
- a sample health care reference letter.
- what to do when you must leave a health care job.
- a health care reference letter activity.

## What Is a Health Care Reference Letter?

A health care reference letter contains statements about your character, abilities, skills, and attitudes. It can be a valuable tool for future health care job interviews. You will use this health care reference letter when applying for future health care jobs by attaching a copy to your employment application, resume, or post-interview letter. You may also want to present your reference letter during your health care job interviews. Always keep your original letter in your portfolio. Distribute copies only.

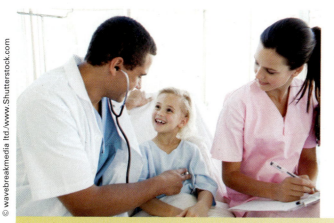
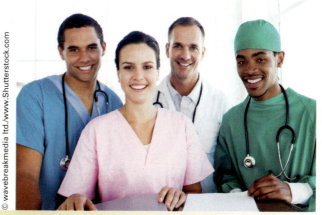

Make sure your reference letter describes your health care professional development.

## How to Obtain a Health Care Reference Letter

Before leaving a health care job, ask your employer or supervisor for a reference letter. Sometimes employers are very busy and they will ask you to prepare your own reference letter, which they may edit and then sign. Usually they will suggest some of the points they would include in the letter. If they do not, ask them if there is anything they would like to say about you in the letter. Do not pass up this opportunity to present the very best side of yourself.

An example of a good health care reference letter is shown in Figure 2.3.1. Notice that the letter is specific about Ken's contributions to the health care facility and mentions positive personality traits.

**FIGURE 2.3.1** Reference Letter

1″ (Line 7)

**ST. CLOUD HOSPITAL
CENTRACARE HEALTH SYSTEM**
1852 Parkway Ave./Reno, NV 89509
(775) 555-8611
2–4S

1″

July 5, 20--

4S

Dear Hiring Manager

2S

**A** Ken Slasor was employed by St. Cloud Hospital for the past two years. As a surgical technologist he displayed excellent skills assisting our surgical team. His timely suggestions for eliminating equipment error during operations were critical to patient welfare.

2S

**B** From the first day Ken quickly became an effective member of our medical team. His job knowledge and consistent effort to learn more about his profession made him a key person on whom we could count. Bottom line, besides being dependable, Ken communicated well with patients and our supervisory medical personnel.

2S

**C** I highly recommend Ken Slasor as a superior surgical technologist. Please call me at (775) 555-8611, ext. 264, if you would like to speak to me directly about Ken's contributions to St. Cloud Hospital.

2S

Sincerely

4S

*Lisa Boyd*

Lisa Boyd
Head Surgical Nurse

1″

| | |
|---|---|
| **A** | Abilities, skills, and accomplishments |
| **B** | Attitude and character |
| **C** | Invitation to reader to call for more details |

You should try to have a reference letter from each of your employers in your portfolio. Do not overlook including a reference letter from a favorite instructor. This reference letter can include your health care knowledge and classroom performance. A reference letter from your extern or intern health care program supervisor can address your on-the-job training performance. A prospective health care employer will look favorably on these types of reference letters. Be sure to thank each person who gives you a reference letter.

Reference letters may not, however, be enough for prospective health care employers. You should also have health care references with whom a prospective employer can make contact. Ask your health care employer to include in his or her reference letter an invitation to readers to call for more details.

# Special Circumstances: When You Must Leave a Health Care Job

Unless you are very lucky, you probably will not always be able to leave a health care job on your own schedule. You may be laid off, downsized, or fired. Here are some suggestions for making the best of these difficult situations.

## What to Do if You Are Laid Off or Downsized

To be *laid off is* to be put out of work through no fault of your own. Frequently, a general layoff is temporary. If you are laid off, you have two choices: wait until your health care job reopens or find another health care job. Before you decide to wait until your health care job reopens, find out what your chances are for being rehired. If you decide to wait until you are called back, plan your time and financial resources carefully.

If you decide to find another health care job, ask your employer for a reference letter. This letter could help you during interviews for your next health care job. Some health care facilities have policies about not giving out references in order to avoid lawsuits. You should have several sources as references.

Being *downsized* means that the health care facility has decided to reduce its labor force. If you are a victim of downsizing, you are unemployed through no fault of your own. You need to look for another health care job immediately.

## What to Do if You Are Fired/Terminated

Being fired is a serious matter. As a reaction to this unpleasant experience, your confidence and self-esteem may suffer, but it is certainly not the end of your working career. There are many reasons a person may be fired. Some common reasons are the following:

- Poor performance
- Poor work habits
- Negative attitude
- Personality conflicts
- Falsifying health care facility documents
- Violation of health care facility policy

## How Can You Get the Best Outcome from Being Fired?

When your health care supervisor tells you that you are fired, ask if you can talk about it. You should try to make the best of this difficult situation. You do not want your leaving to reflect poorly on your next health care job opportunity. Your goal is to try to neutralize the reason you were fired. In the conversation with your health care supervisor, you should:

- Listen carefully to the reason(s) given for the firing.

- Not argue.

- Tell your health care supervisor that you have learned from the situation.

- Point out qualities that you have contributed to the health care position, such as specific work skills or personal qualities.

After you have listened calmly and expressed your intent to make the necessary changes, ask your health care supervisor:

> "If a prospective health care employer should call for a reference, would it be possible for you to give a neutral reason for my leaving?"

The health care employer might be willing to say you were laid off or just making a job change if he or she thinks you have learned and will make an attempt to change. Many health care employers will go along with this line of thought, especially if your conversation was constructive. Most health care employers will not want to destroy a person's future source of income. With the promise of a neutral reference, you can use the agreed-upon reason for leaving on your next health care job application or in a health care job interview.

It is important not to make excuses, to take responsibility for the reason you were fired, and to learn something from the experience. Carefully examine these reasons and ask yourself the following:

- If poor performance was a problem, do I need more medical training?

- Did I not fully understand the health care job requirements when I was hired?

- Did the health care job requirements change?

- Did personality problems affect my work?

- Was compliance to the work schedule a problem?

- Do I need to change certain work habits and attitudes in order to meet the expectations of another health care employer?

You should answer these questions for yourself before you begin your next health care job search.

## What Do You Tell Prospective Health Care Employers?

Should you mention being fired on a health care employment application or during future health care interviews? You, of course, are the only one who can answer this question. Revealing being fired to possible health care employers might not be in your best interests. Many individuals who have been fired simply say that they are making a change in order to pursue a new career opportunity, or that they are seeking employment in a different type of health care facility. If your former supervisor has agreed to a neutral reason for your leaving, you should feel confident in expressing that reason. In most cases, this type of positive comment satisfies the question, "Why did you leave your last health care job?"

A prospective health care employer may find out you were fired in the course of checking your references. If this embarrassing question, "Were you fired?" arises in an interview, you need to answer "yes." If you are not truthful, and you are hired, you could subsequently be fired for providing false information. At this point, what you say and the manner in which you say it are extremely important. You should:

- Handle yourself calmly.

- Be honest and acknowledge your mistake.

- Show responsibility for what happened.

- Avoid blaming your past employer.

Tell the prospective health care employer that you learned a lesson from the experience. You should stress that because of what you learned from being fired, you are now prepared to be a better employee. Your next health care employer may be more willing to give you a chance to move forward if you are sincerely trying to improve your job performance.

## Questions to Answer if You Are Fired from a Health Care Job

Assume that you have been fired from your health care job. Although you regret the health care employer's decision, you agree with your employer's reasoning. From the information you have learned, answer the questions presented here.

1. What actions would you take if you were fired?

_____

_____

_____

_____

2. What questions should you answer for yourself before you look for another health care job?

_____

_____

_____

_____

**3.** What would you say to the health care employer who fired you?

_____

_____

_____

_____

**4.** If fired from a health care job, what reasons for leaving would you place on an employment application?

_____

_____

_____

_____

**5.** What would you say to a health care facility interviewer who discovered that you were fired from your last health care job and asked for an explanation?

_____

_____

_____

_____

_____

## Activity 16

**ACTIVITY
WORKSHEETS**

### Constructing a Health Care Reference Letter

Use your present job or think about a job you have had. It may have been a paid job with a company, work, including internship, for a health care facility, volunteer work, or participation in a class, group, or association. Using the sample health care reference letter as a guide, remove Activity 16 in Section 3, and write yourself a health care reference letter.

After you have drafted your health care reference letter, show it to your instructor for evaluation. Make any necessary corrections. Then key your reference letter and save the final reference letter on the same thumb drive you used to store your resume. Print your final reference letter on the same size and quality paper you used for your resume. Place your printed reference letter in your employment portfolio for future reference.

**PORTFOLIO
UPDATE**

### StudyWARE™ Connection

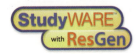

Go to your software and play Hangman to reinforce the benefits of having a reference letter for your next health care job.

# Using the Eight-Step Process to Get and Start Another Health Care Job

Whenever you leave a job, you should follow the first seven steps found in Section 1 of *How to Get a Job in Health Care* to find a new one. Then study Step Eight so your job starts off well. Always update your resume. Even if you left your health care job under unpleasant circumstances, you have probably sharpened current health care skills or acquired new skills and experiences. Get in touch with your network of people. Identify and pursue health care job leads. You may want to practice interview situations to discuss why you left your last health care job. Whatever you do, do not give up. There is a good health care job that is right for you. Your first task is to find it.

## Introduction

The activities in Section 3 of *How to Get a Job in Health Care* are provided to assist you in completing the steps in Sections 1 and 2. These activities provide valuable documents for employment in the health care industry. Be sure to establish an employment portfolio, to use as a file in which to keep your completed activities. Place the completed activities, including keyed resumes and employment letters, in your employment portfolio to reference when you are securing or leaving future health care positions.

The following activities are for the eight steps in Section 1: Getting and Starting a Job in Health Care, and the three steps in Section 2: Leaving a Health Care Job… Gracefully.

### Section 1: Getting and Starting a Job in Health Care

| Step Number | Activity Number | Activity Title |
|---|---|---|
| 1 | 1 | Checklist of Employment Power Words and Phrases |
| 1 | 2 | Writing Health Care Job Objectives |
| 1 | 3.1 | Constructing a Health Care Resume—Standard Resume |
| 1 | 3.2 | Constructing a Health Care Resume—Chronological Resume |
| 1 | 3.3 | Constructing a Health Care Resume—Functional Resume |
| 1 | 3.4 | Constructing a Health Care Resume—Combination Resume |
| 1 | 4 | Constructing a Health Care Reference List |
| 2 | 5 | Writing a Health Care Cover Letter |
| 3 | 6 | Completing a Health Care Employment Application |
| 4 | 7 | Finding Health Care Job Leads |
| 4 | 8 | Researching a Health Care Facility |
| 5 | 9.1 | Answering Interview Questions |
| 5 | 9.2 | Practice Interview Evaluation Form |
| 6 | 10 | Health Care Case Study Questions |
| 7 | 11 | Preparing a Health Care Post-Interview Letter |
| 8 | 12 | Identifying Health Care Personal Qualities |

## Section 2: Leaving a Health Care Job...Gracefully

| Step Number | Activity Number | Activity Title |
|---|---|---|
| 1 | 13 | Health Care Case Study—Decision Time |
| 2 | 14 | Writing a Health Care Resignation Letter |
| 2 | 15 | Health Care Exit Conversation |
| 3 | 16 | Constructing a Health Care Reference Letter |

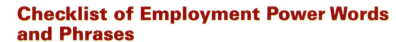

**SECTION 1**   Step 1: Health Care Resume

**Activity 1**

PORTFOLIO
UPDATE

## Checklist of Employment Power Words and Phrases

**Directions:** The following Employment Power Words Checklist contains many assertive and action words and phrases that health care employers want to hear. Use these words and phrases to help write an effective resume, cover letter, employment application, post-interview letter, reference letter, and resignation letter. These power words will help you communicate positively about yourself during your health care interview. When you have completed this to your satisfaction, show it to your instructor for evaluation. Make any necessary corrections. With this activity you establish your employment portfolio. It can be as simple as a file folder. It will contain this completed activity and other important documents, such as your resume and reference list, that you complete in this manual. They all can be used for future reference in getting and leaving a job in health care.

### Employment Power Words and Phrases Checklist

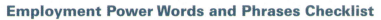

Place a check mark (✓) next to the power words and phrases that you feel describe you best.

I am able to:

| | |
|---|---|
| ___ speak effectively | ___ respect confidentiality |
| ___ be sensitive to feelings | ___ perform with physical stamina |
| ___ analyze situations | ___ set and meet deadlines |
| ___ manage time and resources | ___ respect others impartially |
| ___ follow instructions | ___ organize my work and set priorities |
| ___ motivate others | ___ persistently learn |
| ___ make good decisions | ___ listen attentively |
| ___ be dedicated | ___ be dependable |
| ___ keep up with current changes | ___ take responsibility |
| ___ easily work with others | ___ write accurately |
| ___ use new technology | ___ work well with numbers |
| ___ be accurate | ___ be a problem solver |
| ___ be thorough | ___ teach others |
| ___ be an excellent team member | ___ be flexible |
| ___ work easily with a computer | ___ notice and remember details |
| ___ manage and provide support to others | ___ be a leader |
| ___ follow procedures | ___ read and understand data quickly |
| ___ perform well under pressure | ___ work easily with instruments |
| ___ be goal-oriented | ___ work easily with machines |
| ___ be a self-starter | ___ work independently |

If you have other traits that are beneficial in a health care position, write them on the lines provided here.

_____

_____

_____

Write one phrase that you did not check and would like to improve. Describe how you might develop this quality: _____

_____

_____

_____

Look at the power words and phrases you have checked and those you have listed. Select five that best describe you, and write them here.

**1.** _____

**2.** _____

**3.** _____

**4.** _____

**5.** _____

If you were asked in a health care job interview to describe skills that you would bring to the job, how would you respond? Remember, many of your personal qualities and skills may transfer to health care work and help you succeed in a job.

Answer the question by writing one or two sentences for each of the five power words and phrases you listed. Describe to a prospective health care employer in a job interview how you could demonstrate each quality in the job you are seeking. For example, if you listed "listen attentively," you might say, "I believe that one of my most important skills is my ability to communicate with patients and listen carefully to their needs. I enjoy helping patients feel less anxious knowing they will be cared for well."

**1.** _____

_____

**2.** _____

_____

**3.** _____

_____

**4.** _____

_____

**5.** _____

_____

**SECTION 1**    Step 1: Health Care Resume

**Activity 2**

PORTFOLIO
UPDATE

## Writing Health Care Job Objectives

**Directions:** Write a job objective for each of the medical-related employment ads presented here. Then write a job objective for the health care job you would most like. Write the objectives for a specific health care job title, type of health care work, or a medical-related career goal.

Your health care job objectives should be clearly and concisely written. Use the example of health care job objectives in Section 1, Step 1 as a guide. When you have written your health care job objectives to your satisfaction, show them to your instructor for evaluation. Make any necessary corrections. Place your completed health care job objective worksheet in your employment portfolio for future reference.

Health care position applying for: _____

_____

Health care job objective: _____

_____

_____

_____

**NURSING CNAs
$15/hr**

RNs, LVNs work today!

Apply Online:
Stanfordmedical.net

(510) 555-0166

Health care position applying for: _____

_____

Health care job objective: _____

_____

_____

_____

**MEDICAL**

**Receptionist/ Scheduler** needed to work in our outpatient and hospital-based radiology offices in Alamo and Danville. We offer competitive salary and benefits. Medical experience required. Please fax resume to (925) 555-2424 or e-mail to hbana@bnni.net

Health care position applying for: _____

_____

Health care job objective: _____

_____

_____

_____

Now think of the health care job you want and write a job objective for that position.

The health care position I am applying for: _____

_____

My health care job objective: _____

_____

_____

_____

## SECTION 1    Step 1: Health Care Resume

### Activity 3.1

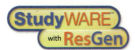

**PORTFOLIO UPDATE**

## Constructing a Health Care Resume— Standard Resume (Practice Sheet)

**Directions:** Gather information about your education and work experience. Complete this outline by writing your resume information on the lines that follow. When you have completed this outline to your satisfaction, show it to your instructor for evaluation. Make any necessary corrections. Next, using this completed outline as a guide, key your resume. Use the sample standard resume in Figure 1.1.2 in Section 1, Step 1 as a reference and spacing guide. Then print your resume following the directions in Section 1, Step 1, Activity 3. Save your resume to your personal thumb drive for easy updating. Keep it updated as you gain experience and education. Place your completed resume in your employment portfolio.

**PERSONAL INFORMATION**

_____
(Name)

_____
(Address)

_____
(City, State, Zip Code)

( )_____        ( )_____
(Telephone Number, Cell Number)

_____
(E-mail Address)

**JOB OBJECTIVE**

_____

_____

**EDUCATION**

(List most recent school first.)

_____
(School Name)

(Year to Present)
_____
(City, State)

_____
(Program)

_____
(Degree)

(Year to Year)
_____
(School Name)

_____
(City, State)

_(Program)_

_(Degree)_

## WORK EXPERIENCE

(List most recent school first.)

(Year to Present)

(Company/Health Care Facility Name)

(Address)

(City, State)

(Job Title)

Responsibilities/Duties: _____

_____

_____

(Year to Year)

(Company/Health Care Facility Name)

(Address)

(City, State)

(Job Title)

Responsibilities/Duties: _____

_____

_____

_____

## MEMBERSHIPS

## HONORS

## SPECIAL SKILLS

## REFERENCES

References available.

**Activity 3.2**

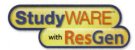

PORTFOLIO
UPDATE

## Constructing a Health Care Resume—Chronological Resume (Practice Sheet)

**Directions:** Gather information about your education and work experience. Complete this outline by writing your resume information on the lines that follow. When you have completed this outline to your satisfaction, show it to your instructor for evaluation. Make any necessary corrections. Next, using this completed outline as a guide, key your resume. Use the sample chronological resume in Figure 1.1.3 in Section 1, Step 1 as a reference and spacing guide. Then print your resume following the directions in Section 1, Step 1, Activity 3. Save your resume to your personal thumb drive for easy updating. Keep it updated as you gain experience and education. Place your completed resume in your employment portfolio.

_____
(Name)

_____
(Address)

_____
(City, State, Zip Code)

(    )_____(    )_____
(Telephone Number, Cell Number)

_____
(E-mail Address)

**JOB OBJECTIVE**

_____

**QUALIFICATIONS**

• _____

_____

• _____

_____

_____

• _____

_____

• _____

_____

• _____

_____

## EDUCATION

_____
(School)

_____
(Degree)

_____
(Month, Year)

## EMPLOYERS

_____
(Month, Year to Month, Year)

_____
(Company Name)

_____
(City, State)

_____
(Job Title)

_____
(Month, Year to Month, Year)

_____
(Company Name)

_____
(City, State)

_____
(Job Title)

_____
(Month, Year to Month, Year)

_____
(Company Name)

_____
(City, State)

_____
(Job Title)

## REFERENCES

References available.

## SECTION 1 | Step 1: Health Care Resume

## Activity 3.3

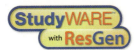

PORTFOLIO
UPDATE

### Constructing a Health Care Resume— Functional Resume (Practice Sheet)

**Directions:** Gather information about your education and work experience. Complete this outline by writing your resume information on the lines that follow. When you have completed this outline to your satisfaction, show it to your instructor for evaluation. Make any necessary corrections. Next, using this completed outline as a guide, key your resume. Use the functional resume in Figure 1.1.4 in Section 1, Step 1 as a reference and spacing guide. Then print your resume following the directions in Section 1, Step 1, Activity 3. Save your resume to your personal thumb drive for easy updating. Keep it updated as you gain experience and education. Place your completed resume in your employment portfolio.

_____
(Name)

_____
(Address)

_____
(City, State, Zip Code)

(____)_____(____)_____
(Telephone Number, Cell Number)

_____
(E-mail Address)

**JOB OBJECTIVE**

_____

_____

**QUALIFICATIONS SUMMARY**

(License and Certification)

- _____

- _____

- _____

- _____

- _____

- _____

- _____

- _____

- _____

- _____

## WORK EXPERIENCE

(List most recent work
experience first)

_____
(Company/Health Care Facility Name/ City, State/ Year to Year)

_____
(Responsibilities/Duties)

- _____

- _____

- _____

- _____

- _____

_____
(Company/Health Care Facility Name/ City, State/ Year to Year

_____
(Responsibilities/Duties)

- _____

- _____

- _____

- _____

- _____

## REFERENCES

References available.

## SECTION 1    Step 1: Health Care Resume

## Activity 3.4

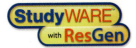

**PORTFOLIO UPDATE**

### Constructing a Health Care Resume— Combination Resume (Practice Sheet)

**Directions:** Gather information about your education and work experience. Complete this outline by writing your resume information on the lines that follow. When you have completed this outline to your satisfaction, show it to your instructor for evaluation. Make any necessary corrections. Next, using this completed outline as a guide, key your resume. Use the sample combination resume in Figure 1.1.5 in Section 1, Step 1 as a reference and spacing guide. Then print your resume following the directions in Section 1, Step 1, Activity 3. Save your resume to your personal thumb drive for easy updating. Keep it updated as you gain experience and education. Place your completed resume in your employment portfolio.

_____
(Name)

_____
(Address)

_____
(City, State, Zip Code)

(     ) _____     (     ) _____
(Telephone Number, Cell Number)

_____
(E-mail Address)

**JOB OBJECTIVE**

_____

_____

**SUMMARY OF QUALIFICATIONS**

(Your Accomplishments/ knowledge)

• _____

• _____

• _____

• _____

• _____

**WORK EXPERIENCE**

_____     _____
(Job Title)                    (Company/Health Care Facility/ Organization Name, City, State)

(Year to Year)     (Responsibilities, Employment Skills)

_____

_____

_____

_____

(Job Title)     (Company/Health Care Facility/Organization Name, City, State)

(Year to Year)     (Responsibilities, Employment Skills)

_____

_____

_____

_____

(Job Title)     (Company/Health Care Facility/Organization Name, City, State)

(Year to Year)     (Responsibilities, Employment Skills)

_____

_____

_____

_____

## EDUCATION

(Degree/ License/Certificate/Credentials, School Name, City, State)

_____

_____

_____

_____

## REFERENCES

References available.

**SECTION 1**    Step 1: Health Care Resume

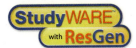

**Activity 4**

PORTFOLIO
UPDATE

## Constructing a Health Care Reference List

**Directions:** Begin this activity by identifying several people whom you may use as a job or personal reference. Then write the reference information on the lines that follow. When you have completed your health care reference list to your satisfaction, show it to your instructor for evaluation, and make any necessary changes. Use the sample reference list in Figure 1.1.6 in Section 1, Step 1 as a guide to create your reference list. Then key your final reference list and save the file on the same thumb drive as your resume. Print your final reference list on the same size, color, and quality paper as your resume. Place your printed reference list in your employment portfolio for future reference.

**REFERENCES of**

_____
(Your Name)

_____
(Name)                                (Title)

_____
(Organization)

_____
(Number and Street Address)

_____
(City)                    (State)              (Zip Code)

_____
(Area Code, Telephone Number)        (Area Code, Cell Number)

_____
(E-mail Address)


_____
(Name)                                (Title)

_____
(Business/Health Care Organization Name)

_____
(Number and Street Name)

_____
(City)                    (State)              (Zip Code)

_____
(Area Code, Telephone Number)        (Area Code, Cell Number)

_____
(E-mail Address)


_____
(Name)                                (Title)

_____
(Business/Health Care Organization Name)

_____
(Number and Street Name)

_____
(City)                    (State)              (Zip Code)

_____
(Area Code, Telephone Number)        (Area Code, Cell Number)

_____

(Name)                          (Title)

_____

(Business/Health Care Organization Name)

_____

(Number and Street Name)

_____

(City)                          (State)                  (Zip Code)

_____

(Area Code, Telephone Number)


_____

(Name)                          (Title)

_____

(Business/Health Care Organization Name)

_____

(Number and Street Name)

_____

(City)                          (State)                  (Zip Code)

_____

(Area Code, Telephone Number)

## SECTION 1    Step 2: Health Care Cover Letter

### Activity 5

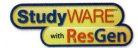

PORTFOLIO
UPDATE

### Writing a Health Care Cover Letter

**Directions:** To complete this activity, first write your practice health care cover letter on this paper. Use the sample cover letters in Figures 1.2.1, 1.2.2, and 1.2.3 in Section 1, Step 2 as guides. Your name, address, telephone and cell number with area code, and your e-mail address need to be shown in the heading to make it easy for you to be contacted. When you have drafted your cover letter to your satisfaction, show it to your instructor for evaluation, and make any necessary corrections. Next, using this completed draft, key your cover letter and save it on the same thumb drive as your resume. Print your final cover letter on the same size, color, and quality paper as your resume. Place your printed health care cover letter in your employment portfolio for future reference.

_____
(Your Name)

_____
(Your Mailing Address)

_____

_____

_____
(Your Telephone and Cell Number)

_____

_____
(Your E-mail Address)

_____
(Date of Letter)

_____
(Name of Person)

_____
(Medical Organization Name)

_____
(Street Address)

_____
(City, State, Zip Code)

_____
Dear

_____
(Purpose of letter)

_____

_____

_____

_____

_____

_____

_____

_____

_____

_____

_____

(Qualifications or reasons why applicant should be interviewed)

_____

_____

_____

_____

(Request for interview)

_____

_____

_____

_____

Sincerely

_____

(Your Signature)

_____

(Your Name Keyed)

Enclosure

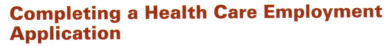

**SECTION 1**   Step 3: Health Care Employment Application

**Activity 6**

PORTFOLIO
UPDATE

## Completing a Health Care Employment Application

**Directions:** Look at the employment applications for ValleyCare Health Center on the following pages (Figure 3.3.1 and Figure 3.3.2). Complete this first one in pencil so you can easily make corrections. Use the sample employment application in Figure 1.3.1 in Section 1, Step 3 as a guide. When you have neatly completed this activity, show it to your instructor for evaluation, and make any necessary changes. Then use your pencil draft, and copy the second employment application in a pen with black ink. Then place it in your employment portfolio for reference when completing employment applications in the future.

**FIGURE 3.3.1** Application for Employment at ValleyCare Health Center (Front)

# VALLEYCARE
# HEALTH
# CENTER

## EMPLOYMENT APPLICATION

ValleyCare Health Center is an equal opportunity employer. This philosophy calls for equal opportunities for employment, training, and advancement regardless of sex, race, creed, color, age, national origin, religion, physical or mental handicap, or genetic information

PRINT CLEARLY

## PERSONAL INFORMATION

DATE _____     SOCIAL SECURITY
NUMBER _____

LAST

NAME _____
LAST                          FIRST                          MIDDLE

PRESENT ADDRESS _____
STREET          CITY              STATE          ZIP CODE

PERMANENT ADDRESS _____
STREET          CITY              STATE          ZIP CODE

TELEPHONE NO. ( ) _____   CELL NO. ( ) _____   E-MAIL _____

FIRST

CAN YOU, AFTER EMPLOYMENT, SUBMIT
VERIFICATION OF YOUR LEGAL RIGHT TO
WORK IN THE UNITED STATES?     CIRCLE ONE:     YES     NO     (IF YES, VERIFICATION
WILL BE REQUIRED)

## EMPLOYMENT DESIRED

POSITION _____        DATE YOU
CAN START _____     SALARY
DESIRED _____

MIDDLE

ARE YOU EMPLOYED NOW? _____     IF SO MAY WE INQUIRE
OF YOUR PRESENT EMPLOYER _____

AVAILABILITY:     DAYS     NIGHTS     PMS     WEEKENDS     FULL TIME     PART TIME

| **EDUCATION** | NAME AND LOCATION OF SCHOOL | DEGREE OR CERTIFICATE OR LICENSE | SUBJECTS STUDIED |
|---|---|---|---|
| HIGH SCHOOL | | | |
| UNIVERSITY OR COLLEGE | | | |
| TRADE, BUSINESS, OR CORRESPONDENCE SCHOOL | | | |

CONTINUED ON OTHER SIDE

**FIGURE 3.3.1** Application for Employment at ValleyCare Health Center (Back)

LIST SPECIAL SKILLS, QUALIFICATIONS, AND PERSONAL QUALITIES THAT APPLY TO THIS POSITION:

_____

LIST WORKING KNOWLEDGE OF: COMPUTER SOFTWARE/EQUIPMENT/LANGUAGES:

_____

LIST PROFESSIONAL ORGANIZATIONS: _____

_____

_____

WORK EXPERIENCE

_____

List all present and past employment, including part-time or seasonal, beginning with the most recent.

| Employer | Employment Dates and Salary | Describe the work you did in detail | Reason for leaving |
|---|---|---|---|
| Name _____ <br> Address _____ <br> City _____ State _____ <br> Phone _____ Supervisor _____ | From: _____ <br> To: _____ <br> Starting Salary _____ <br> Ending Salary _____ | | |
| Name _____ <br> Address _____ <br> City _____ State _____ <br> Phone _____ Supervisor _____ | From: _____ <br> To: _____ <br> Starting Salary _____ <br> Ending Salary _____ | | |
| Name _____ <br> Address _____ <br> City _____ State _____ <br> Phone _____ Supervisor _____ | From: _____ <br> To: _____ <br> Starting Salary _____ <br> Ending Salary _____ | | |

**REFERENCE:**
GIVE THE NAMES OF THREE PERSONS NOT RELATED TO YOU WHO CAN ATTEST TO YOUR EXPERIENCE AND QUALIFICATIONS.

| NAME | BUSINESS NAME/ADDRESS | BUSINESS PHONE | OCCUPATION |
|---|---|---|---|
| 1 _____ | | | |
| 2 _____ | | | |
| 3 _____ | | | |

I AUTHORIZE INVESTIGATION OF ALL STATEMENTS CONTAINED IN THIS APPLICATION. I UNDERSTAND THAT MISREPRESENTATION OR OMISSION OF FACTS CALLED FOR IS CAUSE FOR DISMISSAL. FURTHER, I UNDERSTAND AND AGREE THAT MY EMPLOYMENT IS FOR NO DEFINITE PERIOD AND MAY, REGARDLESS OF THE DATE OF PAYMENT OF MY WAGES AND SALARY, BE TERMINATED AT ANY TIME WITHOUT ANY PREVIOUS NOTICE.

DATE _____ SIGNATURE _____

**FIGURE 3.3.2** Application for Employment at ValleyCare Health Center (Front)

# VALLEYCARE
# HEALTH
# CENTER

### EMPLOYMENT APPLICATION

ValleyCare Health Center is an equal opportunity employer. This philosophy calls for equal opportunities for employment, training, and advancement regardless of sex, race, creed, color, age, national origin, religion, physical or mental handicap, or genetic information

PRINT CLEARLY

## PERSONAL INFORMATION

DATE _____     SOCIAL SECURITY NUMBER _____

NAME _____

LAST                    FIRST                    MIDDLE

PRESENT ADDRESS _____

STREET          CITY          STATE          ZIP CODE

PERMANENT ADDRESS _____

STREET          CITY          STATE          ZIP CODE

TELEPHONE NO. (   ) _____  CELL NO. (   ) _____  E-MAIL _____

CAN YOU, AFTER EMPLOYMENT, SUBMIT
VERIFICATION OF YOUR LEGAL RIGHT TO
WORK IN THE UNITED STATES?     CIRCLE ONE:     YES     NO     (IF YES, VERIFICATION WILL BE REQUIRED)

LAST

FIRST

MIDDLE

## EMPLOYMENT DESIRED

POSITION _____  DATE YOU CAN START _____  SALARY DESIRED _____

ARE YOU EMPLOYED NOW? _____  IF SO MAY WE INQUIRE OF YOUR PRESENT EMPLOYER _____

AVAILABILITY:          DAYS          NIGHTS          PMS          WEEKENDS          FULL TIME          PART TIME

| EDUCATION | NAME AND LOCATION OF SCHOOL | DEGREE OR CERTIFICATE OR LICENSE | SUBJECTS STUDIED |
|---|---|---|---|
| HIGH SCHOOL | | | |
| UNIVERSITY OR COLLEGE | | | |
| TRADE, BUSINESS, OR CORRESPONDENCE SCHOOL | | | |

CONTINUED ON OTHER SIDE

**FIGURE 3.3.2** Application for Employment at ValleyCare Health Center (Back)

LIST SPECIAL SKILLS, QUALIFICATIONS, AND PERSONAL QUALITIES THAT APPLY TO THIS POSITION:

_____

LIST WORKING KNOWLEDGE OF: COMPUTER SOFTWARE/EQUIPMENT/LANGUAGES:

_____

LIST PROFESSIONAL ORGANIZATIONS: _____


_____
_____

WORK EXPERIENCE

_____

List all present and past employment, including part-time or seasonal, beginning with the most recent.

| Employer | Employment Dates and Salary | Describe the work you did in detail | Reason for leaving |
|---|---|---|---|
| Name _____<br>Address _____<br>City _____ State _____<br>Phone _____ Supervisor _____ | From: _____<br>To: _____<br>Starting Salary _____<br>Ending Salary _____ | | |
| Name _____<br>Address _____<br>City _____ State _____<br>Phone _____ Supervisor _____ | From: _____<br>To: _____<br>Starting Salary _____<br>Ending Salary _____ | | |
| Name _____<br>Address _____<br>City _____ State _____<br>Phone _____ Supervisor _____ | From: _____<br>To: _____<br>Starting Salary _____<br>Ending Salary _____ | | |

**REFERENCE:**
GIVE THE NAMES OF THREE PERSONS NOT RELATED TO YOU WHO CAN ATTEST TO YOUR EXPERIENCE AND QUALIFICATIONS.

| NAME | BUSINESS NAME/ADDRESS | BUSINESS PHONE | OCCUPATION |
|---|---|---|---|
| 1 _____ | | | |
| 2 _____ | | | |
| 3 _____ | | | |

I AUTHORIZE INVESTIGATION OF ALL STATEMENTS CONTAINED IN THIS APPLICATION. I UNDERSTAND THAT MISREPRESENTATION OR OMISSION OF FACTS CALLED FOR IS CAUSE FOR DISMISSAL. FURTHER, I UNDERSTAND AND AGREE THAT MY EMPLOYMENT IS FOR NO DEFINITE PERIOD AND MAY, REGARDLESS OF THE DATE OF PAYMENT OF MY WAGES AND SALARY, BE TERMINATED AT ANY TIME WITHOUT ANY PREVIOUS NOTICE.

DATE _____ SIGNATURE _____

**SECTION 1**   Step 4: Finding and Researching a Health Care Job and Facility

**Activity 7**

## Finding Health Care Job Leads

**Directions:** To find health care job leads, record the source you used, and the name of the person who gave you the lead (if applicable), the health care facility name, your contact and their title, the date, telephone number, e-mail if available, mailing address, and important remarks on the forms provided here. The sources you use may include the following ones suggested in Step 4:

| | |
|---|---|
| School Career or Placement Office | Your Professional Medical Association |
| Your Network | Federal Government Job Website |
| Market Survey | One-Stop Career Center |
| Internet | Private Employment Agency |
| Newspaper Employment Ad | Temporary Employment Agency. |

When you have completed your health care job lead information, show it to your instructor for evaluation. Place these contacts in your employment portfolio help with future leads.

PORTFOLIO
UPDATE

### Job Lead 1

Lead Source _____

Name of Person Who Gave You the Lead _____

Name of Health Care Facility _____

Contact Person _____

Title _____ Contact Date _____

Telephone _____ E-mail Address _____

Address _____

City _____ State _____ Zip _____

Remarks _____

_____

_____

## Job Lead 2

Lead Source _____

Name of Person Who Gave You the Lead _____

Name of Health Care Facility _____

Contact Person _____

Title _____ Contact Date _____

Telephone _____ E-mail Address _____

Address _____

City _____ State _____ Zip _____

Remarks _____

_____

_____

## Job Lead 3

Lead Source _____

Name of Person Who Gave You the Lead _____

Name of Health Care Facility _____

Contact Person _____

Title _____ Contact Date _____

Telephone _____ E-mail Address _____

Address _____

City _____ State _____ Zip _____

Remarks _____

_____

_____

## Job Lead 4

Lead Source _____

Name of Person Who Gave You the Lead _____

Name of Health Care Facility _____

Contact Person _____

Title _____ Contact Date _____

Telephone _____ E-mail Address _____

Address _____

City _____ State _____ Zip _____

Remarks _____

_____

_____

**Job Lead 5**

Lead Source _____

Name of Person Who Gave You the Lead _____

Name of Health Care Facility _____

Contact Person _____

Title _____ Contact Date _____

Telephone _____ E-mail Address _____

Address _____

City _____ State _____ Zip _____

Remarks _____

_____

_____

**Job Lead 6**

Lead Source _____

Name of Person Who Gave You the Lead _____

Name of Health Care Facility _____

Contact Person _____

Title _____ Contact Date _____

Telephone _____ E-mail Address _____

Address _____

City _____ State _____ Zip _____

Remarks _____

_____

_____

## SECTION 1 — Step 4: Finding and Researching a Health Care Job and Facility

### Activity 8

PORTFOLIO
UPDATE

### Researching a Health Care Facility

**Directions:** To complete this activity, first select one to three health care facilities you would like to research. Do your research at your school library or career center, your local library, at a health care facility, or on a health care facility Website. Be aware that some health care facilities, especially smaller ones, may not have much information written about them. If that is the case, you could write, telephone, or e-mail the health care facility with your questions. If convenient, you could also visit the facility.

Answer the questions that are provided in this activity for each health care facility you select. When you have completed the research to your satisfaction, show it to your instructor for evaluation. Place your completed research in your employment portfolio. In the future, this activity will help you know how to research medical organizations for important information and know what health care facility questions you need answered before any job interview.

Health Care Facility Name_____

What services does this health care facility provide? _____

_____

_____

_____

_____

What kinds of health care jobs do they have? _____

_____

_____

In what cities does this health care organization have facilities? _____

_____

_____

How large is this health care facility? _____

_____

Is the health care facility growing or shrinking in number of employees? _____

_____

What are the health care facility's plans for the future? _____

_____

Who are this health care facility's competitors? _____

_____

_____

Questions I have about this health care organization: _____

_____

_____


Health Care Facility Name _____

What services does this health care facility provide? _____

_____

_____

What kinds of health care jobs do they have? _____

_____

_____

In what cities does this health care organization have facilities? _____

_____

_____

How large is this health care facility? _____

_____

Is the health care facility growing or shrinking in number of employees? _____

_____

What are the health care facility's plans for the future? _____

_____

Who are this health care facility's competitors? _____

_____

_____

Questions I have about this health care organization: _____

_____

_____


Health Care Facility Name _____

What services does this health care facility provide? _____

_____

_____

What kinds of health care jobs do they have? _____

_____

_____

In what cities does this health care organization have facilities? _____

_____

_____

How large is this health care facility? _____

_____

Is the health care facility growing or shrinking in number of employees? _____

_____

What are the health care facility's plans for the future?_____

_____

Who are this health care facility's competitors? _____

_____

_____

Questions I have about this health care organization: _____

_____

_____

**SECTION 1** Step 5: How to Prepare for a Health Care Interview

**Activity 9.1**

## Answering Interview Questions

**Directions:** To complete this activity, remember to have a particular job and health care facility in mind. Then, using your own words, write answers to each interview question. You may also use the suggested answers in Section 1, Step 5 to help you answer the health care interview questions. When you have completed the answers, show them to your instructor for evaluation. Then work in groups to practice answering the questions with your written replies. Have one person complete Activity 9.2, the Practice Interview Evaluation Form. After the interview, discuss the evaluation results, then switch roles.

Health care position for which I am interviewing:_____

1. Why are you interested in this health care position?

_____

_____

_____

_____

2. We need a reliable person for this health care position. Can we rely on you?

_____

_____

_____

_____

3. What pay do you expect?

_____

_____

_____

_____

4. Why do you want to work for our health care facility?

_____

_____

_____

_____

**5.** Have you had any serious illness or injury that might prevent you from performing your duties in this health care position?

_____

_____

_____

_____

**6.** Do you have references?

_____

_____

_____

_____

**7.** What did you like best or least about your last job?

_____

_____

_____

_____

**8.** Are you looking for a permanent or temporary health care job? Do you want full-time or part-time employment?

_____

_____

_____

_____

**9.** Tell me something about yourself. Why do you think we should hire you for this health care position?

_____

_____

_____

_____

**10.** How well do you work under pressure?

_____

_____

_____

_____

**11.** What are your strengths and weaknesses?

_____

_____

_____

_____

**12.** What are your short-term and long-term health care employment goals?

_____

_____

_____

_____

## SECTION 1    Step 5: How to Prepare for a Health Care Interview

## Activity 9.2

### Practice Interview Evaluation Form

Health care position for which I am interviewing: _____

**EVALUATOR:** Please rate the performance of the person being interviewed. Use the criteria listed below. For each attribute, rate the person on a scale from 1 to 5 as appropriate for the interview (1 is poor, and 5 is excellent). Circle one number. Use the Comments line to make constructive remarks.

| Criteria | Rating |
|---|---|
| 1. Makes eye contact with the interviewer. | 1 2 3 4 5 |

Comments _____

_____

2. Has appropriate posture.                                                      1 2 3 4 5

Comments _____

_____

3. Speaks clearly and is easy to understand.                          1 2 3 4 5

Comments _____

_____

4. Self-confidence while answering the interviewer's question.   1 2 3 4 5

Comments _____

_____

5. Describes skills and abilities in relation to the job.              1 2 3 4 5

Comments _____

_____

6. Has appropriate answers to the questions asked.                1 2 3 4 5

Comments _____

_____

7. Overall evaluation.                                                             1 2 3 4 5

Comments _____

## SECTION 1  Step 6: During the Health Care Interview

## Activity 10

### Health Care Case Study Questions

**Directions:** Carefully review the model health care interview between Jessica Lee and Mr. Kevin Mansell in Section 1, Step 6. Since this is a model interview, you should become very familiar with the answers and practice them before your next interview. When you have completed the case study answers to your satisfaction, show them to your instructor for evaluation. Now answer the following questions:

1. Make a list of six facts that Jessica knows about the health care position after the interview.

   a. _____

   b. _____

   c. _____

   d. _____

   e. _____

   f. _____

2. Make a list of six facts that Mr. Mansell knows about Jessica after the interview.

   a. _____

   b. _____

   c. _____

   d. _____

   e. _____

   f. _____

3. How did Jessica attempt to convince Mr. Mansell that her lack of medical transcription employment was not important in considering her for the job opening?

   _____

   _____

4. In the interview, how did Jessica say that her school classes helped her?

   _____

   _____

For a future interview, tell how your school classes have helped you.

_____

_____

**5.** What was Jessica's answer to Mr. Mansell's question, "Why would you want to work for Danville Health Center?"

_____

_____

How had Jessica prepared for this question?

_____

_____

**6.** What was Jessica's answer when Mr. Mansell asked what she liked best about working for Hammond's Discount Bookstore?

_____

**7.** How did Jessica give a positive answer to Mr. Mansell's question, "Can you describe a stressful situation and how you handled it?"

_____

_____

Describe a stressful situation that you experienced. How did you handle it?

_____

**8.** What answer did Jessica give to Mr. Mansell's question, "What pay do you expect?"

_____

_____

**9.** How does Jessica plan to follow up her interview with Mr. Mansell?

_____

_____

What follow-up technique would you have used? Why?

_____

_____

**10.** Reread the end of Jessica's conversation with Mr. Mansell.

Was it too short?

_____

Was it complimentary?

_____

What would you add or take out?

_____

_____

**11.** If Mr. Mansell should decide to hire Jessica, would you feel he had matched the right person to this health care position?

_____

Why or why not?

_____

_____

_____

_____

## SECTION 1 · Step 7: After the Health Care Interview

### Activity 11

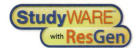

PORTFOLIO
UPDATE

## Preparing a Health Care Post-Interview Letter

**Directions:** To complete this activity, first write your practice post-interview letter below using the sample post-interview letter in Figure 1.7.1, in Section 1, Step 7 as a guide. When you have drafted your letter to your satisfaction, show it to your instructor for evaluation. Make any necessary corrections. Next, using this completed draft, key your post-interview letter following the spacing guidelines given in the sample post-interview letter and save it on the same thumb drive used for your resume. Print your final post-interview letter on the same size and quality paper used for your resume. Place your final keyed post-interview letter in your employment portfolio for future reference.

_____
Your Name

_____
Your Mailing Address

_____
Your Telephone and Cell Numbers

_____
Your E-mail Address

_____
Date of Letter

_____
Name of Person

_____
Title of Person

_____
Health Care Facility Name

_____
Street Address

_____
City, State, Zip Code

_____
Dear

_____
Thank-you and positive comment about interview

_____

_____

_____

_____

_____

_____

_____

_____

Emphasize strengths

_____

_____

_____

_____

_____

_____

_____

Continued interest, additional reasons for hiring, and when and how to contact

_____

_____

_____

_____

_____

_____

_____

Sincerely

Your Signature

Your Name Keyed

## Activity 12

WEBSITE

PORTFOLIO
UPDATE

### Identifying Health Care Personal Qualities

**Directions:** Listed here are words that describe personal qualities that are important in performing many health care jobs. This activity will help you understand which personal qualities relate to your health care job. Follow the steps outlined below to complete this activity. When you have completed this activity to your satisfaction, show it to your instructor for evaluation. Then place it, along with the printed copy of your O*Net OnLine job information, in your employment portfolio for future reference.

First, using the O*Net OnLine printed copy you have of your job title information, go to the "Work Styles" category. Under "Work Styles" there are headings such as: Attention to Detail, Dependability, Concern for Others, Cooperation, Integrity, and Self Control. Read and note the personal qualities that describe each of the headings you find. These are some of the personal qualities that describe what individuals like you, who have this health care job, need to be successful.

Now read this list of personal qualities that health care workers may have. Circle each of the personal qualities on this list that you found for your health care job on your O*Net copy.

#### Health Care Personal Qualities

| | | |
|---|---|---|
| accepting | conscientious | forceful |
| accurate | considerate | friendly |
| adaptive | consistent | gentle |
| alert | controlling | helpful |
| appreciative | creative | honest |
| assertive | decisive | imaginative |
| calm | dependable | independent |
| careful | detailed | innovative |
| caring | efficient | inquisitive |
| cautious | empathetic | logical |
| composed | energetic | loyal |
| cooperative | encouraging | methodical |
| comforting | ethical | motivating |
| committed | enthusiastic | objective |
| compassionate | fair | observant |
| conceptual | flexible | open-minded |

| | | |
|---|---|---|
| organized | reassuring | stable |
| patient | reflective | supportive |
| precise | reliable | sympathetic |
| persistent | respectful | systematic |
| personable | responsible | tactful |
| persuasive | resourceful | thoughtful |
| pleasant | self-confident | thorough |
| positive | selfless | trustworthy |
| practical | sensitive | |
| productive | sincere | |

If there are *other* health care personal qualities that describe your job and *are* listed on your O*Net copy, but *not* listed above, write them on the lines provided here.

_____

_____

_____

Look at the personal qualities you circled and the ones you wrote on the lines above.

Of the personal qualities you have circled or listed, which three do you believe best describe you? These are your strongest personal qualities. Write them on the lines below. Describe how each of these personal qualities is important to you in your health care job.

My health care job: _____

**Personal Quality:**
How it is important to my health care job:

_____

_____

**Personal Quality:**
How it is important to my health care job:

_____

_____

**Personal Quality:**
How it is important to my health care job:

_____

_____

## Activity 13

### Health Care Case Study—Decision Time

**Directions:** Read the following case study on Aaron Rodgers, who wants to make a decision about leaving his health care job. In the space provided, write the advantages and disadvantages of Aaron staying in his current health care position and answer the questions that follow. When you have completed the answers to your satisfaction, show it to your instructor for evaluation and class discussion. Then place this activity in your employment portfolio for future reference.

PORTFOLIO
UPDATE

---

Aaron Rodgers has been employed by Maumee Medical Center, a large health maintenance organization, as a medical assistant for almost three years. At first he was happy with his health care job. He enjoyed his independence and the environment of the health care facility. Now, Aaron goes home some nights with a splitting headache. His doctor recently told him that his blood pressure was up and he should relax more. Aaron's job stress developed when the Maumee Medical Center started making changes in the last year. Aaron has a new supervisor, who often questions how he does things. Worse, one person, who started working there after Aaron, was promoted. Aaron felt he was ready for the assistant supervisor position the person received. Also, the health care facility is much more rigid than when he started. There are more paperwork duties and rules to follow than before. While he is not happy with the work environment, Aaron still enjoys his experience of handling and dealing with a variety of patients. He enjoys having opportunities to attend his health care facility–sponsored conferences and seminars. He is also thinking about becoming trained as an X-ray technician on new, state-of-the-art equipment that has just been installed. Aaron thinks he should just quit, but his living expenses have increased, and his car loan will not be paid off for another year. In two years he will be fully eligible for the health care facility's profit sharing and savings plan.

---

**1.** From the case study, identify at least three advantages and three disadvantages to Aaron's staying in his current health care employment.

|  Advantages of Staying | Disadvantages of Staying |
|---|---|
| 1. _____ | 1. _____ |
| _____ | _____ |
| 2. _____ | 2. _____ |
| _____ | _____ |
| 3. _____ | 3. _____ |
| _____ | _____ |

|              Other Advantages              |           Other Disadvantages           |
| ------------------------------------------ | --------------------------------------- |
| _____   | _____ |
| _____   | _____ |
| _____   | _____ |
| _____   | _____ |
| _____   | _____ |
| _____   | _____ |

**2.** Do you think Aaron should or should not leave his current health care position? Why?

_____

_____

_____

_____

_____

**3.** If you decide he should stay, list three things Aaron could do to improve his health care job situation.

_____

_____

_____

_____

_____

## SECTION 2 | Step 2: The Best Way to Leave a Health Care Job

### Activity 14

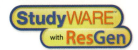

PORTFOLIO
UPDATE

### Writing a Health Care Resignation Letter

**Directions:** To complete this activity, first write your practice health care resignation letter below. Use the sample health care resignation letter in Figure 2.2.1, in Section 2, Step 2 of this manual as a guide. When you have drafted the letter to your satisfaction, show it to your instructor for evaluation. Make any corrections that are needed. Next, using this completed draft, key your resignation letter and save it on the thumb drive used for your resume. Print your final health care resignation letter on the same quality paper used for your resume. Place your printed resignation letter in your employment portfolio for future reference.

_____
Your Name

_____
Your Mailing Address

_____
Your Telephone/ Cell Number

_____
Date of Letter

_____
Name of Person

_____
Title of Person

_____
Health Care Facility Name

_____
Street Address

_____
City, State, Zip Code

_____
Dear

_____
Date of resignation and positive reason(s) for leaving

_____

_____

_____
Appreciation of professional development

_____

_____

Appreciation of fellow employees and health care facility

_____

_____

_____

Sincerely

Your Signature

Your Name Keyed

## SECTION 2  | Step 2: The Best Way to Leave a Health Care Job

## Activity 15

**PORTFOLIO
UPDATE**

### Health Care Exit Conversation

**Directions:** Complete this activity by writing your practice health care exit conversation below. Use the sample health care exit conversation in Section 2, Step 2 as a guide. Notice the positive remarks in this example, and construct your own positive health care exit conversation. Try to make this as relevant as possible to your situation by having in mind a present or past employer. When you have completed your written conversation to your satisfaction, show it to your instructor for evaluation. Make any corrections that are needed. Place your written health care exit conversation in your employment portfolio for future reference.

Notice of Resignation and Reason(s) for Leaving

_____

_____

_____

Positive Comments about Health Care Work Experience (Health Care Facility or Co-workers)

_____

_____

_____

_____

_____

Statement of Health Care Job Skills Learned/Work Habits Improved

_____

_____

_____

Offer to Train Replacement

_____

_____

_____

_____

**SECTION 2**   Step 3: Health Care Reference Letter

## Activity 16

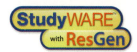

**PORTFOLIO UPDATE**

### Constructing a Health Care Reference Letter

**Directions:** To complete this activity, first write your practice reference letter below. Use the sample reference letter in Figure 2.3.1 in Section 2, Step 3 as a guide. You may want to use the name of your present or a past employer as your reference. When you have drafted the letter to your satisfaction, show it to your instructor for evaluation. Next, using this completed draft, key your reference letter and save the file to the same thumb drive on which you have your resume and other job-related documents. Print your final reference letter on the same quality paper used for your resume. Have your reference person sign the letter, and then place the keyed reference letter in your employment portfolio for future reference.

LINCOLN
MEDICAL CENTER
482 Concord Drive/Lincoln, NE 68502-4901
(402) 555-2888

*Reference letters from employers should be on company letterhead*

Date of Letter
_____

Dear Hiring Manager
_____

Abilities, skills, and accomplishments
_____

_____

_____

_____

_____

Attitude and character
_____

_____

_____

Invitation to reader to call for more details
_____

_____

_____

Sincerely

_____

Signature of Employer

_____

(Keyed)

_____

Name of Employer

_____

Title of Employer